DUDE, WHERE'S MY STETHOSCOPE?

DUDE, WHERE'S MY STETHOSCOPE?
and other stories from the ER

Donovan Gray, M.D.

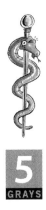

Copyright © 2012 by Dr. Donovan Gray

All rights reserved. No part of this publication may be reproduced, stored in a retrieval system, or transmitted, in any form or by any means (electronic, mechanical, photocopying, recording or otherwise) without the prior written permission of the author.
Printed in Canada

For information about permission to reproduce sections of this book, write to Dr. Donovan Gray:

5grays Publishing
P.O. Box 21106 Charleswood
Winnipeg, MB
R3R 3R2

DISCLAIMER
This narrative is based on real-life events; however, names, ages, genders, diseases, locations and/or dates have been changed in order to protect the privacy of the patients described.

ISBN 9781492818571

Design by Angel Guerra/Archetype
Author photograph by Ruth Bonneville
Illustrations by Dave Whamond
Kudos? Rotten eggs? thegraydude@gmail.com
www.dudewheresmystethoscope.ca

For my four Muses:

Janet *(Sustenance)*
Ellen *(Benevolence)*
Kristen *(Radiance)*
Alanna *(Exuberance)*

Acknowledgments

I would like to thank all the people who have encouraged and helped me with this project:

Birdielyn Gray, Ólöf & Ken Hardy, Joan Hardy & Tim Edginton, Doug & Michelle Chorney, the Sud family, Joanne Mayer, David & Kathy Lanthier, Colin Leslie, Joe McAllister, Dave Whamond, Prakashen & Jenisa Govender, Gregg & Lana Maidment, Theresa & Jerry Cianflone, Danny & Kelly Murray, Jillian Horton, Sonny Cochrane & Ardelle Kipling, Carol-Ann Veenkamp, Angel Guerra, Simon Burns, Sharon Butala, Brian Goldman and Dave Williamson.

A particular thank-you goes to Arnold Gosewich, without whose expertise and guidance this book would never have successfully navigated the convoluted corridors of the publishing world and made its way into your hands.

And, of course, the biggest thanks of all goes to my wife, Janet, for putting up with my impossible work schedules and off-kilter sense of humour for all these years.

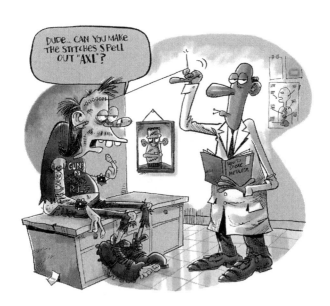

CONTENTS

INTRODUCTION:
10 So What Exactly Made You Want to Become a Doctor?

PART ONE:
Learning the Ropes: Med School and the First Urban ER Year

15 Welcome to the Machine
16 The Peds Ortho Blues
21 Even the Cool Kids Can Fall
24 Dude, Where's My Stethoscope?
28 Fear and Loathing at 3,000 Feet
32 Elementary Questions
34 Life During Wartime
35 The Cleanest Boy *Ever*
37 The Drug Seeker
39 Two-for-One Special in the ER

PART TWO:
Ma & Pa Kettle: The Rural Years

43 Ch-ch-ch-ch-changes
45 Devolution
46 The Big Smoke
50 On-Call Gall
55 It's Got to be in Here Somewhere
57 Semantics
58 Rocky II *(The Sequel)*
60 Alanna's Birth
67 Snip, Snip
70 Last Call
71 Drug Charades!
74 *Haute Cuisine*
77 "I swear, he wasn't breathing!"
78 Rollover Rob *(The Adamantium Man)*

80	Drinking Problem
81	Blood
82	Paralyzed
85	Rick's Tears
89	Parenting 101
90	Adventures in Paralysis *(The Ventilator Blues)*
96	*Koyaanisqatsi (Life Out of Balance)*
96	I, Carnival Duck *(Apologies to I, Claudius)*
102	The Simple Math of Medical Errors
105	Humble Pie
106	Every Breath You Take
108	Thank You
110	Snap!
112	Tough Call
114	So Sue Me
116	3:00 a.m.
117	Carpool Conundrum
122	*Chiaroscuro (Light and Dark)*
123	Lost in Translation
124	Patients Say the Darndest Things!
126	Let's Get Physicals
131	Survey Says . . . .
133	Prescription for Parenting Skills
133	Introspect/*Apologia*
138	Pssst . . . Want to Buy Some Medical Products?
140	Sahara Mouth
141	Beginner's Luck
144	Out-bluffing the Kids
148	*Legerdemain (Sleight of Hand)*
152	Sometimes the Voices Are Real . . . .
153	Status Interrupticus
154	The Call of the Wild *(Sorry, Jack!)*
160	*Tabula Rasa*
161	Some Patients Are Never Ready
163	Shotgun Bubba
164	Disneyfied
164	Slippage

166 My Organic Patient
167 The Wonderful World of Golf
169 Oops!
170 Cancer
171 Betcha Can't Eat Just One
172 Curious George
174 Cerumen
177 For Better or Worse
180 *Prima Donna*
181 Running the Supermarket Gauntlet
186 Rust Ring
188 655: Dead, But Dreaming *(Trapped on Jacob's Ladder)*
190 Time Flies When You're Having Fun!

PART THREE:
There and Back Again: Return to the Big City

193 Should I Stay or Should I Go?
193 "We Put the K in Kwality!"
196 Where's Waldo?
198 Gyne Stretcher at Midnight
199 Lost Soul
201 The Cost of Letting Go
202 Doctor Lockout
204 I Sure Do Love Ol' What's Her Name!
206 Is There a Doctor on Board?
208 Fit for Duty
209 Ode to a Carrot Juice Enema
210 When Your Compassion Runs Out
212 Guilt
213 Time to Go
214 Piece of Cake
215 Skunked
221 For This I Went to Med School? *(Quiet, Sméagol!)*
223 So There You Have It, Folks

INTRODUCTION:
So What Exactly Made You Want to Become a Doctor?

When I was seven I wanted to be a major league baseball player when I grew up. Either that or an astronaut. Doctor was nowhere to be found on my list of potential occupations. The following year my latent allergy genes manifested big-time. Almost overnight I became the undisputed poster boy for atopic disease. After a month or two of watching me scratch, sniffle and wheeze, my mother went out and found us a family physician.

Dr. Grenier was a lanky, middle-aged fellow with curly brown hair and an unruly moustache. He seemed to enjoy making house calls. Every Saturday morning he'd visit our modest little home in Chambly, Québec to give me an allergy shot. Although I wasn't crazy about the injections, I didn't put up much of a fuss because when he was finished he'd always wink and toss me the empty plastic syringe. If he wasn't running too far behind schedule he'd accept my mother's offer of a cup of coffee. While he drank it, he and my dad would sit at the kitchen table and have a spirited debate about whether Rusty Staub and the Montreal Expos would ever manage to climb out of the cellar in the National League East. When the coffee and conversation were finished he'd pack up his mysterious black bag, tell me to be *un bon garçon*, and zoom off in his neon-yellow Citroën.

As I filled the syringe with cherry Kool-Aid and chased my terrified little brother around the house (time for your *needle*, Robin! Bwa-ha-ha-ha!), sometimes I'd concede that although being a baseball player or an astronaut would be amazing, being a doctor might be kind of okay, too.

*

The year I turned 11 my father accepted a job offer from the Ministry of Education in Jamaica. That summer our family packed up and moved from Chambly to a suburb just outside of Kingston. Once the initial culture shock subsided I began exploring my new environment. One good thing about the move was that it allowed me the opportunity to finally meet several family friends and relatives whom I had previously only spoken to on the telephone or seen in photographs. My godfather Maurison was one such person. He was my dad's best friend from back in the Precambrian era when they were both bachelors. Their paths had separated when Maurison immigrated to Germany to study medicine. Upon completion of his studies he returned to Kingston to start a general practice. He could easily have opened his office in an affluent neighbourhood and grown wealthy over time, but that career trajectory held no appeal for him. Instead he set up shop in a desperately poor, underserviced and slightly dangerous part of the city. He worked long hours, coordinated public health outreach programs and allowed his patients to pay whatever they could afford. He didn't get rich, but he loved his work and the community adored him.

Maurison looked after my various allergy-related afflictions, so over the next few years I ended up spending a lot of time in his office. Since I was his godson, no part of the building was considered out of bounds to me. I'd leaf through his illustrated medical textbooks, count the bones in the artificial skeleton hanging in the storage room, marvel at the distorted cortical homunculus figurine and puzzle over arcane pieces of medical equipment in the various cupboards and drawers. The one I liked best was a device similar to an egg timer that he often carried in one of his lab coat pockets. As far as I could tell, its only function was to ring loudly 30 minutes after it was switched on. One day I asked him what it was for.

"Oh that," he grinned. "If I'm running late and I'm about to see a patient who tends to ramble, I turn it on before I go in. When it starts ringing I exit under the pretense of having to take an urgent call from the hospital. It's not exactly kosher, but sometimes that's the only way I can escape from an examination room!"

"Wow," I thought, as I left his office that day, "Life-saving work. Cool gear. A dash of subterfuge. Aside from the lousy hours, medicine's not such a bad gig after all . . . ."

*

When I was 19 my family moved from Jamaica back to Canada. We arrived in Winnipeg a few weeks before I was scheduled to enter university. My grades were excellent, but I had no clue as to what I wanted to study. Education? English literature? Law? In the midst of my tortuous deliberations I got a letter from Paul, a good friend from my high school in Jamaica. He informed me that my old flame was dating a medical student. *What?!* That did it. In the blink of an eye my decision was made – I'd take the prerequisite two years of health sciences courses and then apply to the Faculty of Medicine.

The following essays and anecdotes chronicle some of the experiences I've had over the course of my medical career. It's been a fantastic adventure, and it is still unfolding.

*

P.S. Several years after I graduated from med school I discovered my friend got the story all wrong – the fellow my ex had dated had been studying aviation, not medicine. I'm glad Paul didn't get his facts straight, otherwise right now I'd probably be somewhere up in the stratosphere piloting a 747. And I *really* hate flying.

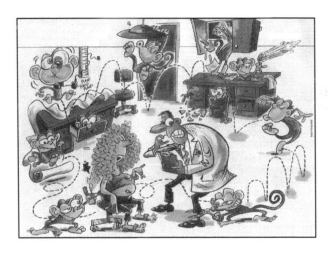

PART ONE
Learning the Ropes: Med School
and the First Urban ER Year

Welcome to the Machine

There is nothing more exciting than opening your mailbox and finding a big, fat envelope from the medical school you applied to. Skinny envelope – not so good. Those contain cachectic little one-pagers that may as well begin, *"Dear John . . . ."* A bulging envelope, on the other hand, means you're in like Flynn. I got mine back in the spring of 1983. At the time my parents were both teaching up in northern Manitoba and my brother had already left for school, so I had to do the Snoopy Dance by myself. Didn't matter. I was still the happiest guy in the world.

Nowadays when I reflect on how cavalierly I approached the entire med school application process I shake my head in disbelief. Not only did I not bother to take any MCAT prep courses, I only left myself enough time to write it once before the application deadline. I elected to apply to a single medical school rather than to the customary five or six. Lastly, I refused to wear a suit to the all-important interview (those were my fractious motorcycling days, and at the time I felt suits were *definitely* not cool). Despite my best passive-aggressive attempts to sabotage myself, I got in. Then the real fun began.

My first inkling I wasn't in Kansas anymore came on the first day of the term when each of our seven lecturers assigned us roughly 25 pages of reading homework. 175 pages wouldn't have been that difficult had we been granted a few days to slog through the material, but they all seemed to expect we'd have everything memorized by the next morning. On day two another 100-plus pages were piled on. And so on. By the end of the first week we were drowning in paperwork. But med school was just getting warmed up . . . .

During the second week we began working in the cadaver dissection lab, or Gross Lab as it was affectionately referred to by our preceptors. I had never even *seen* a human corpse before, never mind taken a scalpel to one. I was so wigged out by the concept that the night before our first trip to the lab I had a nightmare about working down there alone and turning around to find a cadaver sitting up and staring at me. It was like something straight out of *The X-Files*. I woke up in a pool of cold sweat.

The next morning 99 nervous newbie first-year medical students filed silently into the lab. As we answered the alphabetical roll call we were assigned six to a body; three down the cadaver's left side and three down the right. Once we were all in our proper places we were given the order to unzip our respective body bags. When I peeled open our bag the distasteful tang of formaldehyde leapt into the air. Although no one keeled over and face-planted like those poor saps in the opening credits of Quincy, I have to admit we did all take an involuntary half-step backwards before pausing to inspect our cadaver. Approximately 60, male, tall, thin, left forearm anchor tattoo. Dead. A few seconds passed and no one in our group moved forward. After another several seconds I realized what was going on – no one wanted to be the first to touch the body. We eyed each other nervously. Then the fellow next to me leaned over and raised the cadaver's wrist. He furrowed his brows and pantomimed checking for a radial pulse.

"So tell me, Mr. Jones," he said in his deepest baritone, "how long have you been feeling this way?"

We all burst out laughing, picked up our scalpels and got to work.

The Peds Ortho Blues

In the winter of 1985 my classmates and I were turned loose on the unsuspecting wards. At the time we were "baby clerks," fresh out of two years of sitting in our medical school's darkened lecture theatres and still struggling to make sense of the countless thousands of pages of physiological facts floating around in our heads. My own clerkship rotation schedule kicked off with a one-month stint on the notoriously busy pediatric orthopedics service. I wasn't the least bit worried. In fact, I was confident I'd be making more saves than Hippocrates and Grant Fuhr combined.

On the first morning of the rotation I arrived on the ward at 8:30 sharp. A quick search of the area failed to reveal any doctors, so I made inquiries at the nursing station. A harried-looking ward clerk stopped stamping requisitions long enough to inform me the team had finished rounds an hour ago. Since then the house staff had gone down to the ER to see some consults and the surgeon had headed off to the outpatient clinic. I decided to check out the latter.

When I got there I was surprised to find the waiting room already full. Inside there were four rooms. The orthopod saw patients in three of them while the plaster technician applied casts in the fourth. One of the examining room doors was closed. I could hear muffled voices behind it. I walked over to it and was poised to knock when the door suddenly banged open. I was nearly bowled over by a short, 40-ish, balding fellow with thick glasses. He was wearing greens, a lab coat and purple clogs. He thrust his right arm out, shook my hand briskly and said: "Hi, I'm Dr. Stone. You must be my new clerk. Glad to have you aboard! You can just follow me around for now."

Without further fanfare he rushed into the next room, expertly grabbing the file out of the plastic chart rack beside the door as he went by. Upon entry he pulled a small tape recorder out of one of the pockets of his lab coat and proceeded to dictate a note on the child he had just seen. He paused for a second to introduce himself to the new patient's parents and shake their hands. He then resumed dictating. When he was finished, he slipped the tape recorder back into his pocket and nodded at the parents. Thus cued, they launched into a description of their child's problem. Every so often Dr. Stone nodded his head and grunted knowingly. When he figured he had enough to go on he scooted over to the examining table where the little girl was sitting and began twisting her left knee in every possible direction.

"No need to worry," he declared a short while later. "This problem should correct itself as she grows. I don't think she'll require surgery. Please bring her back in six months for a recheck." He fielded a few questions before doing a nimble 180 and blasting out the door, his trusty tape recorder already in hand.

As this pattern was repeated umpteen times over the course of the next two hours, it became excruciatingly clear to me that I knew next to nothing about real-life pediatric orthopedics. Eventually we took a five-minute break while Dr. Stone went down to the operating room to sort out a glitch in his schedule. When he returned he dispatched me to the plaster room to learn some casting skills. The tech was a jovial fellow with a terminal case of verbal diarrhea. He seemed to be hell-bent on giving me the entire two-year cast tech course in an hour and a half. By the time I left the clinic my head was spinning.

After lunch I returned to the ward. There I was introduced to the rest of the peds ortho team: a cranky intern and an even crankier resident. They both looked as though they hadn't slept in weeks. Apparently the service was chronically short of house staff, and this month wasn't going to be any different. The resident divided the ward patients between the intern and me and told us to see them, review their charts and write progress notes. The afternoon passed uneventfully.

At 5:00 p.m. we met to do sign-out rounds. When rounds were completed I picked up my knapsack and walked to the door with a relieved smile on my face. *Survived my first day on the wards! Piece of cake!*

"Where are you going?" asked the resident.

"Home," I answered.

"You can't go home – you're on call tonight. Didn't you see the schedule?"

My smile evaporated.

"No, I didn't. Live and learn, I guess. Who's on call with me?"

"Well, normally we put you newbs on with an intern or a resident, but right now we're so short you're going to have to take call by yourself."

That didn't sound too enticing.

"Who's going to be my backup?"

"Dr. Stone."

"Oh, that's good."

"Not necessarily. He takes call from home, and he doesn't like to be contacted unless it's for something really big."

Oh, crap.

About 10 minutes after they left I was paged to the pediatric ER to see a girl with a broken upper arm. I tried to recollect what the chatty plaster technician had told me earlier about casting a fractured humerus. Something about an army-navy sling with sugar tongs. Or was it sugar buns? Whatever. I doped out a reasonable facsimile and went to town. Putting the contraption on was quite a battle – the child was developmentally delayed and she kept swinging her broken arm all over the place. I could feel the bone fragments grinding against one another whenever she moved. I had to keep reminding myself not to wince. The final product was no Michelangelo, but I was pleased nonetheless.

"Bring her to the fracture clinic next week for a recheck," I said to her guardians in my most impressive doctor voice.

"Why does she need to come back again so soon?"

"Okay, make it a month."

Half an hour later I was back to see a teenage wall-puncher with fractured knuckles. I wasn't sure about the angles the various joints were supposed to be cast in, so I perused the bible – Salter's textbook – and started slathering plaster on. The end result was a hand cast the size of a boxing glove. It was a miracle the guy could lift his arm off the stretcher.

"It'll get lighter when it dries," I chirped optimistically. "Come see us in the fracture clinic in a month."

"That long?" he said dubiously.

"Okay, make it next week."

An hour later emerg called me to see a 9-year-old with a fractured femur. *Geez, isn't that the biggest bone in the body?* I scurried into the ER plaster room to find a stoic but uncomfortable little boy waiting for me on a stretcher. His father lunged out of his chair and shook my hand like I was the Messiah.

"I'm so glad you're here! I'm Mr. Singer and this is my son Jake. The emergency room doctors didn't want to give him anything more for pain until you assessed him."

"Oh. Well . . . ."

"Have you had a chance to look at his x-rays yet? How serious is the break?"

"Er . . . ."

"Is he going to need surgery? Will you have to operate tonight?"

"Um, well, I'm not actually the surgeon. I'm the medical student."

His eyes widened and he gasped. He looked horrified.

"When will the surgeon get here?"

"I'm not exactly sure. They tell me he doesn't come in for every case. How about if I examine your son and then call Dr. Stone to see what he recommends?" Mr. Singer didn't appear to be too thrilled with that plan. His nostrils flared and his eyebrows began to knit together ominously. "I expect he'll come in right away for a major case like this, though," I added hastily.

After the examination I telephoned Dr. Stone. I described the fracture to him and asked if there was anything he wanted me to do before he arrived.

"Oh, I don't need to come in for that," he replied. "Just put him in a Thomas splint and admit him to the ward. I'll look at him in the morning when we do rounds. If you have any trouble with the splint, I'm sure the emerg doc will give you a hand. Good job! See you!"

I returned to the cast room and sheepishly notified Jake's dad that Dr. Stone would not be coming in after all. He was not the least bit pleased. His displeasure bloomed into near-wrath as he watched me fumble around with the splint, trying to figure out how to apply it correctly. Charlie Chaplin had nothing on me. Eventually the ER doctor noticed my unintentional slapstick and came to my rescue. He also ordered more analgesics for poor Jake.

I hadn't even started on Jake's admission paperwork when a razor-thin ER nurse with hair an aberrant shade of red stuck her head in the door and yelled in my general direction: "Hey, ortho! You better not go anywhere – an ambulance is coming in Amber Charlie Three with a girl who just jumped out of a third-storey window. They think she might have a broken back!"

A broken back? What am I supposed to do with that?

Sure enough, a minute later the ambulance attendants came bustling in with a teenager on a stretcher. They had her trussed up tighter than a Thanksgiving turkey – spine board, cervical collar, sandbags, splints, tape and Velcro. The only part of her that wasn't immobilized was her mouth, and it worked fine.

"My neck hurts! My left leg is numb! I have to pee!" she squalled at the top of her lungs.

While I was busy wringing my hands and trying not to hyperventilate, the ER doctor examined her in detail. When he was finished he came over to me and said: "She seems to be stable right now. She's going to need baseline blood work, plus x-rays of her entire spine, pelvis, femurs, ankles and heels. She may also need to go down for a CT scan.

Normally I'd look after everything, but I have to do a lumbar puncture on a septic baby and they tell me another ambulance is on its way in with a kid who's been seizing for 20 minutes. Since this girl's injuries are primarily orthopedic, I'm going to hand her over to you. Call in your staff guy and maybe even neurosurgery if you need backup."

If I need backup?

My new acquisition resumed her litany: "My back is sore! My head hurts! Get me off this board!"

I was in the process of trying to decide whether I should have my brain hemorrhage now or later when the Crayola redhead poked her head through the drawn curtains and bellowed: "Hey, ortho! We have two more consults for you! And that teenager you casted earlier is back with his dad – they're saying his cast is too tight! What the heck kind of cast did you put on his hand, anyway? It looks like a freakin' beach ball!"

I could feel my eyes starting to bug out. I herky-jerked across the room like a defective marionette, scooped up the nearest telephone receiver and dialled Dr. Stone's number. He picked up on the third or fourth ring. I could hear some trippy jazz music playing in the background.

"Hello?"

"I NEED HELP NOW!"

He didn't even ask what the problem was. All he said was, "I'll be there in 10 minutes." And he was.

Even the Cool Kids Can Fall

Mark was a crazy friend of mine back in the early years of med school. He was the most chill guy I'd ever met. The ultimate non-conformist, he did whatever he wanted, whenever he wanted to do it.

On the day of med school interviews, Mark was one of the few applicants who chose not to wear a monkey suit. He showed up at the designated time sporting his trademark handlebar moustache, a couple of earrings, a CAT Diesel baseball cap, a leopard-skin muscle T-shirt, jeans and sneakers. He didn't try to snow the panel with treacle about wanting to save the whales, either. Undoubtedly they found his attitude refreshingly different and he was accepted into medical school.

During our first year Mark continued to be coolness personified. He was a knockout tae kwon do black belt. He dressed like a hardcore punker. He slam-danced to bands like the Dead Kennedys and rode the lightning with Metallica. In addition, he was a bright, energetic and thoroughly likable guy.

Mark would bow to no Moloch. To that end, he quickly worked out a system for not letting medical school take control of his life. This primarily involved studying at home rather than coming to our downtown campus every day for lectures. If he showed up for a lecture and it turned out to be shite he'd usually be able to convince several of us to ditch the class and take off with him. We would invariably end up playing pinball or shooting pool in the student lounge. A couple of times a month our low-life crew would head over to the local watering hole to swill beer and watch strippers. Can you think of a more entertaining way to learn surface anatomy?

Two-thirds of the way into first year, Mark started to run into trouble. His driving became more erratic. His amusing collection of unpaid parking tickets gradually morphed into a serious problem. He found it increasingly difficult to keep up with the demanding med school workload and his grades began to slip. At the end of first year he was told he'd have to write an exam during the summer holidays to determine whether he would need to repeat the year. He hit the books hard and eked out a passing grade.

Unfortunately, things continued to unravel during second year and by the end of it Mark had become visibly disillusioned. He decided to take some time off to travel to the Far East and find himself. The faculty strongly recommended Mark wait until he graduated before embarking upon any long trips, but our turbulent anti-hero had already made up his mind. He bought a backpack and an open-ended ticket and set off for Thailand with high hopes. Nine months later a complete stranger returned.

When Mark got back, the first thing evident was his pierced nose with its diamond stud. But right after that you couldn't help but notice his eyes. They had become ancient. There was a huge emptiness behind them. When he looked in your direction you got the impression he wasn't really seeing *you*, but rather he was staring right through you into some other world. A bleak, unhappy place.

Who knows what he was seeing? He didn't talk much, and when he did his voice was toneless and subdued. He would often start a sentence and then stop halfway through it, as though his train of thought had derailed. Occasionally the old spark would briefly reappear and he'd go on a spiel about something in his usual manic fashion, but before long his words would trail off into silence.

What had happened to Mark in Asia? Rumours began to swirl. Had he gotten into some bad drugs? I don't think so – he had never been into anything heavy prior to the trip. Had mental illness struck? There were whispers of schizophrenia, bipolar disorder, PTSD . . . . No one but Mark knew the whole story, and he wasn't telling. Each time we tried to probe deeper to find out what had gone wrong he retreated behind a stony wall of silence. That September Mark joined the medical class one year behind us to resume his training, but within a few months he had washed out miserably. He took some more time off to regroup and tried again the following year. Things went better that time and he was able to stay afloat long enough to complete the theoretical portion of the curriculum and advance to the dreaded wards.

I don't know how things are now, but back then the wards of our teaching hospitals were harsh environments where only the strong survived. Every four to eight weeks medical students were tossed into a new subspecialty ward populated with its own unique mixture of complex patients, overworked nurses and terse staff physicians. You had to land on your feet, integrate seamlessly with the new team and quickly learn the ropes. No one was assigned to hold your hand. No one wanted to hear about how sleep-deprived you were. Nobody was even remotely interested in the fact that studying for the mandatory bimonthly exams while working almost every day (in addition to being on call for 24 hours every three days) was nearly impossible. Even well-balanced, mentally healthy students often cracked under the intense pressure. Mark didn't stand a chance. He went down without a trace.

The last time I saw him was about 20 years ago. I used the phone book to figure out where he was living. It turned out to be his mother's place in the north end of town. When I telephoned no one picked up, but I really wanted to see him so I took a chance and drove over to the address anyway.

I knocked on the door for nearly five minutes before Mark shambled out. He had gained a lot of weight. His skin was pasty. The cool hair, leather jacket and easy grin were gone, as was his confidence. He looked haunted. It was painfully obvious he was embarrassed about the way things had turned out for him. During the course of the conversation I mentioned the Asia trip a couple of times but it seemed to make him edgy, so I backed off. We sat on his front steps and small-talked about music, motorcycles and the good old days for awhile.

Needless to say, it was an awkward reunion. I didn't stay long. On the way home hard tears stung my eyes.

Dude, Where's My Stethoscope?

By 1989 I had completed my basic four-year MD degree and was more than halfway through an additional three-year residency in family and emergency medicine. That summer I took a break from the crucible of my ER and ICU rotations and travelled to McMaster University in Hamilton, Ontario for a leisurely month of training in dermatology. The specialist to whom I was assigned was a leader in the field, so I got a lot of great hands-on experience.

One Friday morning I was busy working in his outpatient clinic. It was nearly noon and I was getting hungry. I had just finished dictating what I hoped would be my last note before lunch when Dr. Crowe tapped me on the shoulder. I groaned inwardly when I realized he was holding a chart in each hand.

"Two patients left," he said. "One's new and the other's a follow-up. Which would you prefer?"

"I'll see the new one."

"Okay. Come and get me when you're done." He passed me the chart and ambled off.

The referring physician's letter indicated the patient had an eight-week history of an itchy, red rash that hadn't responded to steroid creams and two courses of Nix. Seemed straightforward enough. I opened the door and walked into the treatment room.

There were three people inside – a man, a woman, and a baby. I estimated both adults to be in their mid-30s. The woman looked downtrodden. The man was short, stocky and unfriendly.

"We've been sitting here waiting for half an hour!" was his opening gambit.

"Sorry, sir. The clinic was unusually busy this morning."

"Are you the specialist?"

"No, I'm Dr. Gray, a family medicine resident." I extended my hand; he didn't take it. "I'll see you first, then Dr. Crowe will be in," I continued.

"More delays," he grumbled.

"Where's your rash?" I asked.

"All over." He peeled off his tank top to reveal a spotty, red rash covering most of his torso.

"How long have you had it?"

"Doesn't it say in the damned letter?"

I gave up on trying to elicit any further information and proceeded to examine him. The rash looked like scabies to me, but his family physician had already treated him for that without success. I cobbled together a differential diagnosis and told him I'd return with the specialist shortly.

"Better not be long! Doctors aren't the only people who have things to do, you know!"

I located my preceptor and reviewed the case with him.

"I've got an extremely prickly 34-year-old man with a two-month history of an itchy rash all over his body. He looks like a pizza with legs. His family doctor thought it was either eczema or scabies, but Betaderm ointment and two rounds of Nix haven't helped," I reported.

"What else is on your differential?"

"Pityriasis, contact dermatitis, vasculitis, erythema multiforme, flea bites . . . ."

"Let's go see."

"Hi, Mr. Grendel, I'm Dr. Crowe. I've been hearing about this unusual rash of yours. Would you mind taking off your shirt again so I can have a look at it?"

"How many times does a guy have to get undressed before he gets a diagnosis around here?" he carped under his breath as he wriggled out of his wife-beater.

Dr. Crowe studied the dappled rash for a few minutes. He looked fascinated.

"We'll need to do a biopsy," he concluded. "Dr. Gray here will do the procedure. I'll stop by and have a look when he's finished."

Great....

I earmarked a fresh lesion to excise and opened a biopsy kit. Before donning sterile gloves I took off my stethoscope and placed it on a nearby countertop so it wouldn't get in the way.

The procedure went well. While I dictated my note at the main desk, the patient and his family packed up and left.

Approximately 10 minutes later I realized I wasn't wearing my stethoscope. I checked my knapsack and searched the reception area. There was no sign of it.

"Could you have left it in one of the treatment rooms?" the clinic nurse asked. Of course! I went back to retrieve it. It wasn't there. It took me a minute to figure out what had happened.

"That last patient took it," I said.

"Who?" asked the nurse.

"The guy I did the biopsy on. Which way did he go?"

"I think I overheard him saying something to his wife about catching a bus."

"Where do they live?"

She checked his file. "Stoney Creek."

"Where's the bus stop?"

"You're going after them? Are you out of your mind?"

"They swiped my stethoscope!"

She gave me directions.

They weren't there. According to the schedule on the wall, their bus wasn't due for another 45 minutes. Judging by the size of my patient's belly, he didn't miss too many meals. I headed for the cafeteria.

It was lunchtime and the place was packed. After a couple of minutes of searching, I spotted them eating at a table near the centre of the room.

There were two large plastic bags on the floor at their feet. I circled in from behind, cleared my throat loudly and said: "Excuse me; I think you have something that's mine."

Mr. Grendel spun around. He didn't look the least bit intimidated. Very bad sign.

"What did you say?"

"Hi, I'm Dr. Gray, remember? I think you may have accidentally taken my stethoscope."

"I didn't take any stethoscope," he bristled.

I made another attempt to give him a graceful out.

"Sir, I think it's possible that when you packed your things it may have ended up in one of your bags by mistake."

He detonated. "I didn't take your goddamn stethoscope, and I resent what you're implying!"

Suddenly we were at the epicentre of a rapidly expanding shockwave of silence. Within a few seconds every conversation in the room had ceased. A thousand pairs of eyes locked onto us. I wasn't wearing my name tag or my lab coat, so I'm sure half the crowd must have thought I had just escaped from the psych ward.

I glanced down at the pair of plastic bags on the floor. Several thoughts flashed through my mind. How sure was I he had stolen it? If he did steal it, which bag was it in? I had a 50 percent chance of guessing right. If I searched the wrong bag first, he'd kick up such a fuss I'd never be able to get anywhere near the second bag. How much trouble would I be in if I guessed wrong? Apology-sized trouble? Lawsuit-sized trouble? Should I just cut my losses and walk away? Just then an image of him gloating and strutting popped into my head. It was more than I could stand. I grabbed the bag closest to me and ripped it open.

I didn't see my stethoscope, but the bag was filled to the brim with miscellaneous articles. In for a penny, in for a pound . . . . I started tossing the bag's contents onto the table. A chorus of gasps rang out. Someone dashed to a nearby telephone and called security. I didn't care anymore; I was determined to see this thing through to the bitter end. I continued hauling stuff out of the bag at a furious pace – chips, cigarettes, matches, gum, magazines, Kleenex, Pepsi, Kool-Aid, Carnation formula, diapers, baby wipes . . . .

My stethoscope was at the very bottom of the bag.

Fear and Loathing at 3,000 Feet

In May of 1990 I was in the final stages of my medical training. One evening a fellow resident named Raoul and I were hanging around the cafeteria at St. Boniface Hospital in Winnipeg.

"Hey, Donovan, take a look at this," he said, pointing to a new notice on the bulletin board. It was a sign-up sheet for a one-day skydiving course. Raoul was excited. He figured it would be the ultimate adventure. As for me, I wasn't so sure. I'm deathly afraid of heights, so naturally I had some problems with the concept of leaping out of an airplane at an altitude of 3,000 feet. For the next two weeks, Raoul badgered me incessantly: "Come on, don't be such a wuss! Sign up with me! It'll be the experience of a lifetime!" Eventually I caved in and added my name to the list of thrill-seekers.

As the jump date drew nearer I began to have second thoughts. What the devil had I gotten myself into? The sign-up sheet seemed to leer at me every time I walked by it. *"Pssst! Schmendrick!"* it would whisper sibilantly. *"Is your life insurance policy up to date? Heh-heh-heh . . ."* I was sorely tempted to scratch my name off, but pride prevented me. Would John Wayne have chickened out before *The Alamo*? Hell, no!

On the morning of our jump class I awoke with a colossal knot in my stomach. "Maybe we'll get rained out," I told myself hopefully. When I opened my curtains, brilliant sunlight streamed in. So much for divine intervention. I got dressed and phoned Raoul to see if he needed a ride to the drop zone.

"Hurro?" he mumbled. What was he doing sleeping in on the morning of our big adventure?

"Rise and shine, buddy! Need a ride?"

"Ride?"

"To the drop zone. You know, for today's skydiving lesson."

"Kaff-kaff! I won't be able to make it today, Donovan – bad cold. *Kaff-kaff!"*

Those were without a doubt the lamest coughs I had ever heard.

"Gee, you looked fine yesterday. When did you get this cold?" I asked suspiciously.

"*Kaff-kaff!* Last night. Very bad cold. Sore throat, too! Sorry, gotta go take some cough medicine! Good luck!" He hung up.

I gnashed my teeth all the way to the drop zone.

The No-Frills Jump School was located on a weedy lot 53 miles west of Farmville. It consisted of a tiny prefab trailer and one fly-blown porta-potty. I counted 18 people – 16 students plus a pair of instructors named Daniel and Lucy.

"Where's Raoul?" a colleague from the hospital inquired when I joined the group.

"Bad cold. *Kaff-kaff!*" I replied.

Daniel overheard our exchange and smiled knowingly.

"You'd be surprised how often that happens," he said. He then turned to Lucy and asked, "Where's Fudge?"

"I think he's sleeping in the back of the trailer again."

"We should probably start. Would you mind waking him up?" Daniel blew a whistle to get our attention. "Okay troops, gather round! Fudge is going to be your primary instructor today. He'll be starting shortly. He's a Class One Skydiver with more than 2,000 jumps under his belt. Pay close attention to what he says – your lives may depend on it!"

Just then the trailer's side door creaked open. We all turned to get our first glimpse of the man upon whom our lives would depend.

Fudge was a squat, 30-something fellow with a thatch of matted brown hair and a seedy-looking five o'clock shadow. He was wearing wraparound mirror shades, a tie-dyed T-shirt, fraying shorts and flip-flops. He looked vaguely disoriented. Several seconds elapsed, during which he gazed up at the sky while absentmindedly scratching an armpit. Finally he opened his mouth to speak.

"What day is it?"

Despite our initial misgivings, Fudge turned out to be an excellent instructor. He spent the first couple of hours teaching us the basic rules of skydiving. Among other things, we learned that since we were beginners our canopies would be rigged to automatically deploy a few seconds after we exited the plane. All we had to do was relax and enjoy the ride. Once we got closer to the ground one of the instructors would communicate with us via walkie-talkie to help us steer the parachute safely into the landing area. The whole thing sounded preposterously easy. I began to wonder why I had allowed myself to get so worked up about it. *I should have done this a long time ago! Maybe I should look into bungee jumping, too* . . . . Fudge interrupted my ambitious daydream.

"Hey, Gray, wake up. Now for the fun part, everyone! I'm going to tell you about everything that can go wrong while you're in the air." *Uh-oh*. "Here's an example," he continued. "Every now and then some poor fool gets tangled in the lines of his chute. When that happens, you fall faster than a cannonball. Any of you happen to remember what terminal velocity is?" My stomach lurched. I scanned my fellow jumpers. They all looked like they were about to spew. "120 miles an hour," he said. "Pretty fast, eh? That doesn't leave you with much time to react, so listen up!"

We listened.

An hour later the plane went up with Daniel and three very nervous-looking jumpers. The rest of us watched as the single-engine Cessna climbed to the proper altitude and levelled out over the jump zone. A tiny speck appeared in the plane's doorway. Moments later the speck dislodged and a white parachute blossomed above it. We all cheered like hillbillies at a graduation. A few minutes later the plane circled back and the process was repeated. The third time around, however, the speck at the threshold didn't move. We turned to Fudge.

"Choked," was his simple explanation.

"What happens now?" I asked.

"Daniel will probably give the jumper one more chance," he replied. Sure enough, the plane turned around and passed over the drop zone again. Despite our shouted encouragement, the jumper remained frozen in the doorway. Fudge shook his head sadly. "There's one or two in every class." As the plane began its descent, Fudge handed me a parachute. "Put this on," he said. "You're in my group, and we're going up next."

It was cold and noisy in the airplane. There were no seats behind the cockpit, so the other two jumpers and I sat with our backs pressed against the hull. Fudge lay on his side reading a dog-eared science fiction paperback novel. As the plane ascended, I tried to remember everything he had taught us. I couldn't seem to recall much more than the bit about getting tangled in the suspension lines of the chute, though. Come to think of it, what were we supposed to do if that happened? Oh yeah, "cut away" the main parachute, free fall until we were no longer entangled and then activate the reserve chute. Did screaming like a schoolgirl come before, during or after those manoeuvres? Just then, one of the other jumpers nudged me with her knee. I looked up to see Fudge standing by the door.

"Door!" he yelled over the racket of the engine.

"What?" we yelled back in unison.

He threw the door open.

A tremendous roar filled the plane. I could barely hear myself think. Fudge motioned for me to approach. Although every cell in my body begged me to ignore him, I got up and walked stiffly to the doorway. He surveyed my parachute one last time and then pointed at the footpegs welded to the frame just outside the door. We had practiced standing on them earlier in the day, but that had been on *terra firma*. Circumstances had changed considerably since then. When I leaned out of the plane to step onto the first peg, the wind buffeted me with incredible force. Struggling for balance, I put my left foot on the peg and looked back at Fudge. He smiled broadly. Encouraged, I planted my right foot on the second peg and glanced back again. This time he gave me the A-OK sign and shouted, "Jump!"

*Who, me? You have **got** to be kidding.* I stared down at the ground. It was a billion light-years away. The farmer's fields below were the size of postage stamps, and the roads were thinner than strands of spaghetti. Meanwhile, the howling wind continued to tear at me and screech in my ears. I looked longingly at the interior of the plane. *Sanctuary*. Fudge gave me the thumbs up sign and hollered again for me to jump. I didn't budge. We stared at each other for what seemed like eons. At last he motioned for me to climb back inside. The look of disappointment on his face was unmistakable. Somehow it served to galvanize me. I sucked in a huge breath and vaulted into thin air.

If my life were a cartoon, the thought bubble above my head as I plummeted earthward would have contained nothing more than a giant exclamation mark. My first coherent memory after my frantic leap was the loud snap of the chute opening. After that, the only sounds were the muted drone of the Cessna in the distance and the occasional rustle of the canopy above me. It was strangely peaceful, drifting lazily a quarter of a mile above the prairie. It was also electrifying. I had my next jump date planned long before my feet touched the ground.

Elementary Questions

The summer I completed my medical training I landed a job as an emergency room physician at the Misericordia General Hospital in Winnipeg. One day my mother asked if I'd be willing to come to her elementary school during Career Week to speak about health care. I told her I'd be delighted.

I assumed I'd only be talking to one or two classes, but when I got there the principal apprised me I'd be addressing the entire school and escorted me to the gymnasium. It was packed with kids, all of whom were sitting on blue gym mats and chatting noisily. The principal stepped up to the podium, motioned for the students to be quiet and introduced me. I then launched into a kid-friendly description of my life as an ER doc. When I was finished, I asked if there were any questions. Two dozen hands shot up. I pointed to a boy in the centre of the crowd. He leaped to his feet.

"How old are you?" he queried.

"I'm 29."

"What kind of car do you drive?" he continued.

"Um, a Toyota MR2."

"Is that a sports car?"

"Yes."

"What colour is it?"

"Dark blue."

He grinned and sat down, apparently satisfied with my answers.

I nodded at a tiny girl in the front row who was desperately waving her hands in the air.
"Is Mrs. Gray really your mommy?" she asked.
"Yes, she is."
"Is she nice at home?"
"Yes, she's very nice."
She smiled and sat down.

I pointed to a boy who was wriggling around on his mat like a worm.
"What would you like to know?" I inquired.
"Can I go to the bathroom?"
"Okay."
He sprinted out of the gym.

I made eye contact with a girl near the back of the room. She squealed with delight and jumped up.
"I have a cat named Trixie!" she proclaimed triumphantly.
The audience went *berserk*.
"I have a dog named Rover!"
"I have a goldfish named Gipper!"
"We had a bird, but it died!"
"We're getting a salamander next week!"
"My dog just had puppies!"
"QUIET PLEASE!" yelled the principal. "No more talk about pets! Does anyone have any questions about *hospitals* or *medicine* for Dr. Gray?"

Silence.

Approximately 15 seconds later a solitary hand went up.
"Yes?" I asked cautiously.
"My grandfather lives in Nova Scotia!" *Uh-oh* . . . .
"We went to Disney World last summer!"
"I like Donald Duck!"
"My mommy just had a baby!"

"My dad thinks our cat might be pregnant!"
"Trixie has orange fur!"
"CHILDREN, PLEASE!" screeched the principal.

It was the longest 20 minutes of my life!

Life During Wartime

What can I say about ER work? It's exhilarating, terrifying and hilarious, all at the same time. Like a handful of other strange professions (for some reason law enforcement and stunt acting come to mind) it's impossible to predict what you'll end up seeing over the course of your day. The only thing you can be reasonably sure of is that at some point during each shift you'll run into something you've never laid eyes on before. Sure, there are a number of common ailments that trundle through those annoying sliding doors on a regular basis, but the red neon *Emergency* sign out front also seems to be a magnet for the bizarre. For example, yesterday I treated a woman who had been bitten on the cheek by a horse. Hmm, a horse bite in the middle of the city. Now there's something you don't see every day!

The typical shift in your average urban ER is fairly busy. For starters, you generally have anywhere from 15 to 30 patients tucked under your wing at any given time. It's a heterogeneous group populated by the "worried well" at one end of the spectrum and the seriously ill at the other. Your job as an ER doc is to figure out what's wrong with each patient as quickly as possible and then either fix them or relay them on to someone who can. As you work through each individual's problems you also need to keep updating your mental tally of where all your other patients are in their respective diagnostic workups. Depending on each person's description of their symptoms, their physical findings, the results of any tests ordered, and your instinctive gut feeling, certain illnesses move up or down their list of conceivable diagnoses. Once you've decided on the most likely culprit you can commence treatment and begin working on disposition. Walk-ins, crawl-ins and ambulance drop-offs add new patients to the already volatile mix every few minutes. If anyone in your flock takes a sudden nosedive you need to immediately drop everything and divert your full attention to the new priority. It's not that uncommon to be hastily summoned to the stretcher or bedside of an unfamiliar patient who is only a few heartbeats away from death. In those cases you don't have the luxury of being able to obtain a detailed history and perform a thorough examination to help shape a logical working diagnosis. Instead you have to immediately shift into *augenblick* mode and initiate potentially life-altering treatments based solely on a brief gestalt impression. It's like going from zero to warp speed without even having time to buckle in.

Imagine doing all of this in a cacophonic environment full of telephones ringing, faxes printing, monitors alarming and dozens of people laughing, crying, yelling, cursing, complaining, wheezing, coughing, bleeding and vomiting. I keep picturing some poor slob in a white lab coat juggling 20 buzzing chainsaws while balancing on a tightrope suspended above a shark-infested pool. Who could resist a job like that?

The Cleanest Boy *Ever*

Last Wednesday the ER was a non-stop frenetic cabaret of diseases of every genre. Around 2:00 in the afternoon one of the nurses handed me a chart and said: "I think you should see this one next." A cursory review of the triage note revealed my next patient to be a four-year-old boy named Simon who was presenting with a rash. *Meh.* What's so exciting about that?

I walked into the cubicle and came face to face with Lobster Boy. This poor little tyke was P.T. Barnum sideshow material. His entire body was covered in a brilliant red, swollen rash, and he was scratching like there was no tomorrow. Each time his nails scraped across his skin, huge welts bubbled up almost immediately. I had to force myself not to gawp.

"How long has he been like this?" I asked his mother.

"It started this morning, doctor."

"This looks like an allergic rash. Does he have any allergies that you're aware of?"

"No."

"Has he been in contact with anything different lately? Food, clothing, detergent, medication?"

"No."

"Nothing at all that might have irritated his skin?"

"Not that I can think of."

I couldn't make sense of it. Allergic rashes as startling as this one usually have a readily identifiable precipitant. Examining him didn't reveal any further clues. I asked his nurse to start an IV and administer some corticosteroids and antihistamines. Two hours later he was looking and feeling much better. I decided to allow him to go home on oral medications, provided his mother promised to bring him back in the morning so I could recheck him.

The next day it was his dad who accompanied him. Once again he was covered head to toe in the same horrific scarlet rash. I asked his father if he could think of anything his son might be reacting to.

"Well, I suppose he could be allergic to those magic markers he was playing with yesterday," he speculated. "He got marker all over his body – his arms, legs, face, belly . . . everywhere! The rash started about an hour after that."

"Ah, that's probably what triggered it," I said with satisfaction. Another mystery solved.

"I don't really see how, though," he continued. "He's played with those markers lots before, and besides, the ink wasn't on his skin for very long. The minute my wife saw what a mess he was she marched him straight up to the bathroom and washed it all off."

"Hmm," I said. "Perhaps it's not the markers, then. Could it be the soap she used that irritated his skin?"

"Oh, she didn't use soap, doc."

"What did she use?"

"Fantastik."

"She used *Fantastik?*"

"Yeah."

"Are you talking about the spray-on cleaner? The stuff you clean countertops and stoves with?"

"Yeah, that's it. She sprayed him down in the bathtub and then scrubbed the marker off with a rag. That stuff really works!"

"That stuff is corrosive! It dissolves glass!"

"Hey! Maybe that's why he's been so itchy!"

The Drug Seeker

The first two lines of the triage note on my next patient indicate he wants a prescription refill. *That sounds like an easy one.* Scanning a bit further down I see the word "painkiller." *Uh-oh.* Next comes the word that throws up more red flags than a parade of matadors: "OxyContin." My heart sinks. I compose my face into something appropriately neutral and walk into the cubicle. Not too far in, mind you – I like to have an unobstructed escape route in situations like this. Just in case.

Patient X looks pretty much like I expected. He's in his late 20s with grubby jeans, a frayed black leather jacket and tattoos crawling up his neck. He also has the obligatory "OZZY" tattoos on the knuckles of both hands. I make a mental note to get myself an incredibly original masterpiece of body art like that in the near future. I'm sure it'll turn me into an unstoppable babe-magnet. What cute chick can resist a guy with "OZZY" tattooed across his knuckles?

"Hi Mr. Piltdown. I'm Dr. Gray. How can I help you this evening?"

"I'm in some serious pain, man." *Hmm . . . .*

"Where is your pain located?" *Please don't tell me "everywhere."*

"Everywhere." *Damn, I asked you not to tell me that . . . .*

"What do you usually take for it?" *Surprise me and say Advil!*

"OxyContin." *Oy vey . . . .*

"That's a pretty strong painkiller. Have you tried anything else for your pain?" *Like maybe heroin?*

"I'm allergic to everything else." *Wow, what are the odds?*

"Who usually gives you your prescriptions?" *A guy in a trench coat?*

"Dr. Feelgood at the health clinic in Buffalo Groin, Saskatchewan. I just got off the bus from there and they can't find my suitcase. It had a six-month supply of my pills in it." *They lost your luggage on the bus? Really? When did Air Canada join the bus industry?*

"What other pills did you lose?" I really shouldn't ask that, but sometimes I can't help but be curious as to how far they'll go with a story that's already more improbable than anything Lewis Carroll ever wrote.

He lights up. He senses a patsy!

"Uh, just my sleeping pills and my Ritalin and my nerve pills and . . . ." *And a partridge in a pear tree?*

When I was younger and more foolhardy I used to tell these critters I had some difficulty believing their sketchy stories and was not comfortable filling their Fantasy Island drug wish lists for them. That usually spawned a whine-fest that would inevitably degenerate into either grovelling or death threats. Once I was rooked into calling someone's out-of-province doctor to verify his story. His girlfriend's dog had eaten his pills, as I recall. I wonder how it got the cap off? Must have been related to Lassie.

"Hello?" I began.

"I told you man, quit bugging me! I'll have your money by next week at the latest!"

"Um, is this (416) 867-5309?"

"Oh, sorry dude, I thought you were someone else! Wazzup?"

"My name is Dr. Gray and I'm looking for a Dr. Jenny."

The person at the other end covered his receiver for a moment and gave a few phlegmy coughs. When he started speaking again, his voice had magically descended an octave.

"Hi, this is Dr. Jenny speaking."

"Never mind." *Click!*

Trial and error has led me to an expedient solution to these encounters: "I'm sorry, but I don't prescribe OxyContin to any emergency room patients ever, and I don't make any exceptions to that rule." The vast majority of miscreants seem to accept this. I guess they can tell when the jig is up. Oh well, all in a day's work in the ER. I wonder who's behind the next curtain?

Two-for-One Special in the ER

It was another barmy Monday morning in the department. I picked up the next chart and reviewed the triage note. Mrs. Stewart, an 85-year-old woman with a rash. I knocked on the door and entered.

An elderly, blue-haired woman was seated on the stretcher. There was also a woman in her mid-50s standing in the far corner of the room. I nodded at the younger woman before turning to face my patient.

"Hi, Mrs. Stewart. My name is Dr. Gray."

"What?"

"I said my name is Dr. Gray."

"You made a special tray?"

"MY NAME IS DOCTOR GRAY!"

"Oh, hello Dr. Gray. Please call me Grace. Would you like to see my rash?"

She lifted the back of her shirt to reveal a diffuse, non-specific, red rash. Damned if I knew what it was.

"How long have you had this rash?"

"What?"

"I SAID, HOW LONG . . . . Never mind." I addressed the younger woman. "Do you know how long she's had this rash?"

"I'm sorry, doctor, no."

"Is she on any medications?"

"I don't know."

"Has she ever had a rash like this before?"

"I really have no idea."

I was beginning to develop an irresistible urge to roll my eyes.

"In what way are you two related?"

"We're not."

"Oh, are you just a friend?"

"I've never met her before in my life."

"What?! Then why are you both in the same examination room?"

"I'm not sure, doctor. Half an hour ago a nurse brought me here and told me to wait. A few minutes ago a different nurse brought her in. I think maybe someone made a mistake."

Good thing Mrs. Stewart hadn't come in to get her hemorrhoids checked!

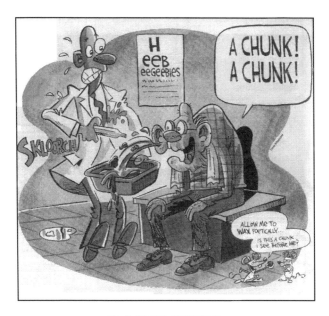

PART TWO
Ma and Pa Kettle: The Rural Years

Ch-ch-ch-ch-changes

In the fall of 1990 my good friend Barb the hairdresser announced she had found the perfect girl for me.

"Yeah, right, Barb," I replied dryly. I'd witnessed some of her previous matchmaking attempts. Not good.

"No, trust me, you'll like this girl! She's really cute and she's got a great sense of humour!"

"Okay, if you say so. What does she look like?"

"Five-foot-four with light brown hair and greenish eyes."

"What does she do?"

"She's an elementary school teacher."

"Sounds promising. What's her name?"

"Janet."

After a few phone calls, Jan and I scheduled a blind date at a nearby Perkins restaurant. The day before we were to meet she came down with a wicked flu. She considered cancelling, but ultimately curiosity got the best of her and she decided to proceed. Aside from her having shaking chills (plus Barb and my buddy Raj unexpectedly sliding into our booth halfway through the meal to mooch some fries and inquire how the date was going), everything went pretty well. We agreed to continue seeing each other.

Meanwhile, back at the ranch, I had come to the conclusion that although I enjoyed working as an ER physician in Winnipeg, I wanted to see what life was like on the other side of the urban/rural divide. Several telephone calls and reconnaissance trips later I accepted a position as a family doctor in a small town in northern Ontario. I shipped a few moving boxes, loaded up my MR2 and headed east in July of 1991.

Making an abrupt transition from a city with a population of 600,000 to a remote hamlet of 6,000 is much like doing the legendary Polar Bear Dip – extremely shocking at first (what do you *mean* there's no Starbucks here?), but then you quickly grow accustomed to it. Then you die of hypothermia. Kidding!

My new gig was a bona fide cradle-to-grave family practice.

Technically it was a solo practice, but I shared ER call and hospital responsibilities with a congenial group of four other family doctors plus a general surgeon. On a typical weekday I would do rounds on my hospital inpatients early in the morning, perform a couple of minor procedures in the emergency department, and then go to my office for a full day of scheduled appointments. When the office wrapped up I would usually return to the hospital briefly to check on my inpatients' progress and review the results of any tests I had ordered earlier. On weekends I'd do my regular hospital rounds first and then spend some time at the local nursing home.

Being responsible for my own inpatients was a deeply rewarding experience, but I won't pretend it was all rainbows and lollipops. For one thing, it meant visiting the hospital 365 days a year unless I happened to be out of town. In addition to commanding a significant chunk of my time, it paid poorly. Despite these drawbacks, there was one very big plus: it allowed me to care for my patients when they needed me most, i.e., when they were sick enough to warrant hospital admission.

Every Wednesday and some weekend days I'd be on call for the ER for 24 consecutive hours. In order to accommodate my ER obligations, my receptionist always booked a lighter office on Wednesdays. This allowed me time to shuttle back and forth between my clinic and the emergency department. The ER tended to be reasonably quiet between 6:00 and 8:00 p.m., so most evenings I'd be able to sneak back to my apartment for supper and a power nap. After that I'd return to the ER and see outpatients until midnight.

The void between midnight and 8:00 a.m. was highly unpredictable and ran the gamut from wonderful to bloody awful. On a good night there'd be no outpatient visits after midnight and I'd be able to get a solid six or seven hours of shut-eye. More often than not, though, people would continue trickling into the department well into the wee hours and my sleep would get hopelessly fragmented. Once in a while I'd get no sleep at all. That gets old *very* fast. It's hard to face the new day when it feels like your head is screwed on backwards.

Aside from missing the action at my old ER in Winnipeg, I was pretty much hooked on my new job right from Day One. There was something immensely satisfying about sending an acutely ill patient from my office to the ER, meeting them there to start treatment, admitting them to the medical ward, rounding on them daily until they recovered and then having them follow up with me back at the office. It was like being an office-based practitioner, an ER physician and a hospitalist all rolled into one. Of course, it's not like I invented that particular enterprise. Most rural (and some urban) generalists have been playing endless variations on that theme ever since Og fell off the first stone wheel and got rushed to the Healing Cave back in 20,000 BC.

Jan and I conducted a long-distance relationship during my first year in Ontario. In July of 1992 we tied the knot and she joined me in my northern adventure.

Devolution

For the first few months after we got married, whenever I was telephoned at home in the middle of the night to go see patients in the emergency department Jan was the epitome of concern. The instant I hung up she would ask me if I had to go in. I'd fill her in on the details as I stumbled around in the dark looking for my clothes. Before I left she'd always say she hoped it wouldn't be long before I was back. When I eventually returned home and crawled under the covers she'd wake up and murmur something appropriately sympathetic in my ear. Ah, those were the days.

As time passed she gradually stopped asking what I was being hauled out of bed to go and see, but she never failed to say, "Do you have to go in, honey? That's too bad." It became a comforting little ritual.

One night I answered the phone at 3:00 a.m. and glumly listened to the ER nurse explain that she needed me to come see some intoxicated yo-yo who was going to require a truckload of stitches. When I hung up Jan rolled over and said, "Do you have to go in, honey?

That's too . . . *zzzzzzzzz* . . . ." As I lumbered out the door I thought, "Uh-oh. Things are definitely slipping."

After that she completely quit waking up for those maddening nocturnal phone calls. I can't really say I blame her – it's probably a sanity-preserving defence mechanism. It certainly preserves her sleep! You could nuke the house next to ours and she'd snore right through it, guaranteed. Some nights I'm recalled to the emergency department three or four times after midnight. Our alarm clock invariably goes off 20 minutes after I've limped into bed for the final time. Jan usually sits up, stretches luxuriously and announces, "What a great night! You didn't get called once!"

"Great night," I croak incoherently.

A few days ago our prehistoric bedroom telephone finally gave up the ghost, so we replaced it. The new phone rings like a klaxon from hell. Last night I was on call. This morning Jan didn't look quite as well-rested as she usually does.

"I don't like that new telephone," she complained. "It woke me up!"

I had to work hard to keep the grin off my face.

The Big Smoke

Not long after we moved to northern Ontario, Jan and I decided to spend a romantic weekend in Toronto. We planned to fly out after work on a Friday evening and attend *The Phantom of the Opera*, then spend the next day shopping. Saturday night we'd have supper at a cozy restaurant. On Sunday afternoon we'd pack up and fly home.

First we made our flight and hotel arrangements. Next we phoned the theatre to purchase tickets. They cost a small fortune, but we'd heard so many wildly enthusiastic reviews about the show we would have gladly paid double the asking price.

The last thing we needed to organize was our Saturday night soirée. Being recently displaced prairie folk, neither of us had the faintest idea where to go in Toronto for a good meal. We solicited advice from our co-workers and one of Jan's colleagues recommended a restaurant he and his wife liked. Jan asked if I'd need to wear a suit or jacket and was assured dress pants with a shirt and tie would be more than sufficient. We called the restaurant and made reservations for 7:00 p.m. on the Saturday.

A couple of weeks later we packed our bags and left for the airport to begin our much-anticipated weekend in the Big Smoke.

After checking into our hotel we spruced up a bit and caught a cab to the theatre. The lobby was packed with excited people. Through one of the doors nearby I glimpsed a portion of the stage as well as the first few rows of seats. I surveyed our tickets: row K, centre. *This is going to be great - 11 rows from the stage!*

We joined one of the queues and slowly inched our way to the nearest door. I handed the usher our tickets. He looked at them, frowned deeply and passed them back to me.

"Is something wrong?" I inquired.

"Sir, these are for row K, upper balcony. This entrance is for the seats on the main floor." He said "upper balcony" like it was some kind of STD.

I quickly re-examined the tickets. Of course he was right.

"Which line should we be in?" I asked.

"Over there." He pointed to a long line at the far end of the lobby. Jan and I mumbled apologies and walked over to the proper line-up. Eventually we made it to the balcony. I looked down at the stage and was disappointed to see the view wasn't that great. *Oh well, 11 rows from the front of the balcony will still be okay.*

When we got to row K I motioned to my wife and started to edge in.

"Wait a minute, this isn't right," said Jan. "This row is full."

"Really?" I backed out.

"Look," she continued, her eagle eyes fixed on the dark nether regions at the rear of the theatre. "Right now we're in the main balcony. Our seats are in the *upper* balcony!"

I thought back to what the usher downstairs had said. Jan was correct. Row K? More like K2! Our seats were going to be so remote, we'd need Sherpas to find them. We steeled our jaws and continued on our quest.

A couple of postal codes later we arrived at row K in the upper balcony. It was one row from the wall at the very back of the theatre. The only people behind us were a few pimply high school kids. They were busy having a lively discussion about the latest Guns N' Roses album. I turned my attention to the stage. From our vantage point it was about the size of a shoebox. A well-decorated shoebox, but a shoebox nonetheless.

The show began. The people onstage looked like ants. Singing ants! What a concept! But why were they so fuzzy? It suddenly occurred to me that in our haste to get to the show on time I had left my glasses back at the hotel.

"I can't see a thing!" I complained to no one in particular.

"Shh!" the high school students chorused.

A few minutes later an usher came by hawking programs. I was tempted to ask him if he also sold high-altitude oxygen bottles, but I knew Jan would slap me silly if I did.

"Do you sell binoculars?" I asked.

"Yes, sir," he replied. "Only $15 apiece."

"I'll take a pair, please." He took my money and ran.

I inspected my new purchase in the half-light. It looked like something you'd get with a McHappy Meal. When I removed the shrink wrap, one of the eyepieces fell off and rolled down the aisle. A Good Samaritan picked it up and returned it to me. I jammed the plastic lens back into place and tried focusing on the stage. If anything, the el cheapo binoculars made it look even farther away. Now the people were no bigger than grains of sand. Singing grains of sand! Gosh, what'll they think of next?

"Hey man, binocs. Cool! Can I try?" asked one of the acne victims behind me.

I tossed the useless binoculars over to him.

"You can keep them," I grumbled. I closed my eyes and settled in for a several-hundred-dollar nap.

The next day we went shopping. I like shopping about as much as the next guy – which is to say, not at all. I basically spent most of the day muling Jan's multiple purchases around the mall. When I started getting blisters on my palms I pleaded for mercy and escaped back to the hotel. Jan returned a few hours later. Her Visa card was so hot it glowed.

Later that evening we started getting ready for our dinner date. At 6:55 a cab dropped us off at the restaurant. As we hung up our coats we agreed we were definitely indebted to Jan's colleague for his tip. The place looked classy and the food smelled delicious.

I walked up to the maître d' and said, "Hi! We have a seven o'clock reservation." He stared at me intently, much like a scientist studying an unusually freakish lab specimen. *Uh-oh.* "Under Gray," I added nervously. He cleared his throat, but didn't say anything. The suspense was gruesome. "Is there some kind of problem?" I finally blurted out.

"Oh no, not at all," he said. "But perhaps *monsieur* would like to wear . . . *zis?*" He reached into a nearby closet and pulled out a threadbare brown corduroy jacket. I recoiled in horror. *Oh, no.* The house jacket – the jacket loaned to charity cases who have the gall (or stupidity) to show up at formal restaurants in inappropriately casual attire. I briefly wondered what Quincy scribbles on his coroner's report when someone dies of embarrassment.

I was about to politely decline his offer and slink out of the place like a mangy cur when three couples sauntered in and lined up behind us, effectively blocking our escape route. I noted miserably that each of the men was wearing a high-end Harry Rosen suit. I recognized the cut because I happened to own one. The problem was that these guys were wearing theirs, whereas mine was hanging uselessly in a closet about 800 kilometres away.

"Sh-sh-sure, I'll wear the jacket," I stuttered. I motioned for him to pass it to me. I was hoping to get it on before anyone else noticed some jackass had tried to defile the dress code.

"Let me help you weeth zat, *monsieur*," he oozed. He then proceeded to hold the arms out for me. I tried not to flinch as I slid my arms in. Behind me I heard one of the Rosen triplets gasp. My cheeks started burning. I snuck a peek at Jan. She looked ill. I finished wriggling into the jacket and straightened up. It was about three inches too short at the wrists. *Hey, look at me – I'm Jethro Bodine!* I had a frightening vision of the maître d' poking around in his carnival closet of terror for a jacket that would fit me better while more and more guys straight off the cover of *GQ* joined the line-up behind us.

"Fits great," I squeaked. "Where do we sit?" Jan and I marched to our table in lockstep. I was certain everyone we passed was gaping at me and whispering, "Is that guy really wearing the house jacket? What's this place coming to? Let's get the hell out of here!"

The food tasted like sawdust.

On-Call Gall

"Once more unto the breach!"

– King Henry in William Shakespeare's
The Life of Henry the Fifth

It's Saturday morning in the ER. I'm about to emerge from my foxhole at the main desk and go on point again. *Born to Cure* . . . .

My first patient of the day is Rocky. He moved to our little duckburg only a few weeks ago, yet he's already racked up an impressive number of alcohol-related ER visits. Rocky lives at "no fixed address" and his home telephone number is "not applicable." This time he's been delivered to us because someone found him crawling around on his hands and knees trying to round up a herd of invisible bugs. I guess everyone needs a hobby. I drain the last of my Tim Hortons coffee, rrroll up the rim (please play again!) and walk over to his cubicle.

Rocky is horizontal on the stretcher. He's a dishevelled-looking fellow in his late 50s. His salt-and-pepper hair shoots out wildly in all directions and he's sporting a week's worth of gnarly stubble. It looks like his nose has been broken a few times. He's heavily doused in that best-selling cologne, *Eau de Stale Booze*. I think he's sleeping.

"Hi Rocky, I'm Dr. Gray."

No response.

"Wake up, Rocky."

He yawns widely and rolls onto his left side. *Ack! Plumber butt much?*

"Rise and shine, Rocky!"

His eyes pop open.

"Whaddayawant?" he grunts. Communication! Hey, now we're getting somewhere. Things are looking up already.

"My name is Dr. Gray. I'm here to see if you're okay. Are you able to sit up?"

Sitting up doesn't pose much of a challenge to most people, but the Rock Man makes it look like it should be included in the decathlon. He plants his elbows firmly by his sides and starts throwing his head forward in a series of jerky attempts to lift his torso off the stretcher. At the same time his legs scissor up and down vigorously. I fail to see how that's going to help the situation. Perhaps Mission Control sent different messages to the upper and lower halves of his body. After about half a minute of flailing he manages to get himself upright.

"Thanks, Rocky. Now I'm going to – "

"Wait!"

"What's wrong?"

"I think I'm gonna be sick!"

"Hang on, I'll get you a basin right away!" Too late – he leans over the wastepaper basket beside his stretcher and does a humongous technicolor yawn: *"Huuurrrraaaalp! Huuurrrraaaalp!"*

There's no sign of blood in the stuff coming up. Big Macs and Pop Tarts, yes, but blood, no. I hand him some towels and canvass the area for a basin.

Does everyone else's workday begin like this?

While an aide cleans up Rocky, I proceed to the next cubicle. In addition to looking like he's just been keelhauled, patient number two is wearing the same cologne as Rocky. Talk about bad luck. This isn't going to be another one of those days, is it?

"Hi, I'm Dr. Gray. How can I help you this morning?"

"I wanna go to detox. I don't have any money, so I'll need a ride, too."

"Okay, we'll see what we can do. When was your last drink?"

"Last night."

"How much did you have?"

"Lots."

"What were you drinking?"

"Lysol and Orange Crush."
"Anything else?"
"Shaving cream."
Mamma mia.

I ask switchboard to contact the intake worker at the nearest available detox centre. Rocky's still barfing up a storm, so I order some IV fluids, Gravol, Valium and thiamine for him before moving on to the third patient. According to the chart, his name is Harley Wayne Gacy. If he's not a serial killer, I'll eat my socks.

"Hi Mr. Gacy, I'm Dr. Gray. That's a very interesting Charles Manson T-shirt you're wearing! Who would have guessed that chainsaws could be so versatile? So, how can I help you today?"

"I need prescriptions for OxyContin, Talwin and Ritalin. And something for my nerves, too. And my parole officer says I have to get these disability pension forms filled out right away . . . ."

Ay, caramba!

My fourth patient presents with a stellate scalp laceration sustained in a booze-induced inward pike off the back of a moving pickup that occurred sometime around midnight. I'm surprised he waited so long to come in - it looks like an asteroid collided with the back of his skull. I give him a complimentary reverse yarmulke and get busy with my suture gear. While I sew him up we listen to the not-so-soothing strains of Rocky repeatedly breaking the 11th Commandment *(Thou Shalt Not Upchuck on the Floor of the ER)*. Half an hour later my crash test dummy is looking human once again. Antibiotic dressings, a tetanus shot and a trip to the radiology suite follow in short order. Not long after that he's exiting stage left. Goodbye Mr. Bloody-Head! No more Olympic asphalt-diving, please! I catch up on my charting and order some IV Maxeran for Rocky.

The receptionist drops another fresh batch of outpatient charts on the ER desk and whispers, "Incoming!" That instantly triggers a harrowing flashback to the time I travelled up the Nung River deep into the heart of Cambodia in search of a brilliant yet almost certainly insane colonel who . . . wait a minute – that was Benjamin Willard, not me. Oops. Sorry about that, folks. Anyhow, the triage note on patient number five reveals he's here today because for the past few months he "just hasn't been feeling quite himself." I know from previous ER encounters that he has a tendency to ramble. This time I'll try to take control of the interview by avoiding open-ended questions.

"Mr. Filibuster, I'm going to ask you a series of questions and I'd like you to just answer yes or no, okay?"

"Okay, doc."

"Have you lost any weight recently?"

"When I was a young 'un living down in Oklahoma back in the Dirty Thirties . . . ."

Can I get a swig of that grape Kool-Aid?

Patient number six:

"Hi, I'm Dr. Gray. How can I help you today?"

"I'm from out of province and I've run out of my birth control pills. Can you give me a refill?"

"No problem. What are they?"

"I'm not sure. Something-21."

"Most of the brands come in packs of either 21 or 28."

"Actually, it might have been Something-28."

Swing low, sweet chariot . . . .

Patient number seven is another prescription refill. The last one was a bit of a gong show, but I'm confident things will go more smoothly this time.

"I'm Dr. Gray. How can I help you?"

"I'm here in Canada on vacation and I've run out of my pills. Can I get some refills?"

"Sure. What medications do you take?"

"I don't know the names."

"Did you bring your bottles with you?"

"No, but I can tell you what the pills look like. There's four white ones, a pink one and a wee little yellow one."

Just take me now, Lord . . . .

Despite having an entire pharmacopoeia at my disposal, Wookiee-like noises continue to emanate from Rocky's cubicle. Eventually I throw in the towel and admit him to the medical ward. The rest of the morning continues on in a similar vein. The afternoon's no prize, either. Around suppertime the nurse supervisor informs me the waiting room is finally empty. Thank God! I was about to change my name to Sisyphus. If I'm lucky, things will stay quiet for a little while. I go home to eat with Jan.

By the way, we never say the Q-word out loud in our department. Every ER worker on the planet knows the instant you make a comment about how quiet it is, a jumbo jet full of ventilated preemies will crash land in your staff parking lot. Probably right on top of your car. That's just the way ER karma rolls.

It is now the witching hour. I'm two-thirds of the way through my 24-hour shift. I think I've treated close to 20 people since I got back at 8:00 p.m. Thankfully, I'm down to the last one. According to the triage note, she's a previously healthy 60-year-old who has been experiencing minor cold symptoms for a week. Her vital signs are all normal. Hmm. Something tells me this case isn't going to make it onto *House*. Oh, well. One last person to see, and then I get to crawl into bed for a while.

"Hello, Mrs. Coryza, I'm Dr. Gray. How can I help you tonight?"

"Well, I've had this runny nose and cough for a week now, so I figured I should come in and get checked."

"Have you had any fever?"

"No."

"Have you been short of breath?"

"No."

"Are you coughing up any sputum?"

"No."

"Any other symptoms?"

"No."

"What made you decide to come in tonight?"

"I just thought it was about time I got some penicillin for it."

Her examination is completely benign. Since I know what she is expecting from this visit, I carefully explain to her why using antibiotics to treat viral upper respiratory tract infections is not appropriate.

She takes a moment to mull it over, then adroitly changes her tack.

"Can I have a chest x-ray, then?" She doesn't need that either, but since she obviously has no intention of leaving this department empty-handed, it's a compromise I can live with. I write up the requisition.

"The x-ray department's closed now. Come back on Monday morning and they'll do it then."

As I turn to leave she says: "You know, my son should probably see you, too."

I'm crestfallen. More business. Precisely what I do not need at this hour of the night. I don't recall seeing anyone else in the waiting room, though.

"Where is he?"

"At home. Can you stay here while I go and get him?"

"Well, that depends. What's wrong with him?"

"He was in a car accident."

"A car accident? What time did it occur?"

"Oh, it didn't happen today; it was about a month ago."

"A *month* ago?"

"Yes. His chiropractor says he's got whiplash, but I think we should get another opinion."

"You want a second opinion on a Saturday at midnight?"

"Yes, I'm wondering if maybe he should be getting some other type of treatment."

There are a number of ways I could respond to this request, but most of them would probably earn me a stern reprimand from the College of Physicians and Surgeons.

"Why don't you bring him in on Monday morning when you come for your chest x-ray?" I suggest sweetly.

"Will you be here Monday?" she asks.

"Yes."

"Okay, that sounds good! Good night, doctor. By the way, you should try to get more sleep – you look really tired!"

It's Got to Be in Here Somewhere

Recently a middle-aged woman took a tumble while jogging on a dirt road. She fell with her arms extended, so her palms and wrists took the brunt of the impact. In ER lingo that mechanism of injury is known as

FOOSH, or "fall on outstretched hand." Hey, don't look at me – I'm not the one who comes up with these half-baked acronyms. Anyway, after going home and removing as much of the gravel from her wounds as she could, she presented to our emergency department. Once I was satisfied there were no other significant injuries I applied a topical anaesthetic gel to her abrasions and scrubbed all the dirt out.

"How's that?" I asked her when I was finished.

"Much better, although it feels like there might still be something in here," she said, pointing to the middle of her left palm.

"Okay, I'll send you over for an x-ray."

Fifteen minutes later I went to the radiology department to look at her films. To my chagrin, there was a pebble-sized object in the centre of her left hand. It appeared to be right on the surface of the skin. How the dickens could I have missed such an obvious foreign body? I returned to the ER with the x-rays and carefully reassessed her hand, but I couldn't find the offending piece of gravel. After a brief discussion we decided our only option was to go in and retrieve it.

Using her films as a map, I infiltrated her left palm with local anaesthetic, made an incision and started looking. No mysterious particle popped into view. I did some blunt dissection. Nothing. I extended the incision radially and continued the search. Nothing but blood. Several minutes passed. Where the hell was it? Every so often my patient would ask, "Find it yet?"

"Not yet, but it's got to be in here somewhere."

After what seemed like an eternity, one of the x-ray techs walked into the room.

"Oh, there they are," he said. "I've been looking for these films all over the place. The radiologist wants to read them before he leaves."

"Could you please ask him if he'd mind waiting for a couple of minutes? I'm using them to help me locate this foreign body."

"What foreign body?"

"The one in her palm," I replied, and pointed it out on the film.

"Oh *that*," he said. "Didn't you get our last memo? We're not using the old arrow-shaped marker to show the spot where the patient has the foreign body sensation anymore. The new marker looks just like a little pebble."

Semantics

A while back I saw an ER patient who was complaining of a persistent cough. It appeared to be nothing more than the common cold, but because it had been going on for a few weeks I elected to send him for a chest x-ray. Once the film was processed I went over to the radiology department to look at it. It was completely normal - no pneumonia, cardiomegaly, congestive heart failure, pleural effusion, pneumothorax or anything else of significance. I went back to the patient's cubicle to wrap up the interview.

"Well, Mr. Kowalski, I don't see anything on your chest x-ray."

"Nothing at all?"

"That's right."

"Okay. Thanks anyway, doc."

I thought he looked at me a little strangely as he left, but I figured I was just being paranoid. I moved on to the next patient.

An hour later I was back in the radiology suite reviewing another film when one of my colleagues showed up. He pulled out the chest x-ray of the patient with the cough I had seen earlier.

"I already looked at that one," I said. "It's normal."

He seemed taken aback.

"What did you say to him?" he asked.

"I told him I didn't see anything on his x-ray."

He started laughing.

"What's so funny?" I asked.

"He called me at my office in a big panic saying he had just had an x-ray at the hospital but the doctor who ordered it didn't know how to read it."

"What made him say that?"

"You told him when you looked at his x-ray *you didn't see anything*."

Needless to say, ever since that day I've changed the way I tell patients their x-rays are normal.

Rocky II *(The Sequel)*

It's yet another Saturday morning and I'm back for more punishment in the ER. Where did all the people in the waiting room come from? Five minutes ago the joint was empty. Maybe spontaneous generation does exist after all.

My leadoff patient is none other than the infamous Rocky. Once again he's toxic and on the verge of hurling. Whenever he shows up like this I usually end up admitting him for a day or two to help him dry out. Things are a little different today, though – there are only two empty beds left in the entire hospital. If I admit him to one of them I'll be snookered if I need beds for sicker patients later on in my shift. To the best of my knowledge, Rocky has never had any potentially dangerous alcohol withdrawal problems such as the DTs or seizures. After careful consideration I make an executive decision to turf him to a detoxification centre. I ask the ER charge nurse to have switchboard locate the closest detox centre's intake worker.

"Aren't you forgetting something?" she asks.

"What?"

"They won't want to take him the way he is now."

True enough. Detox centres don't like their alcoholics drunk and barfy; they like them dry and stable. Most of them will only take "clients" who have been alcohol-free for at least a couple of days.

"Yeah, I know that."

"So how are you going to convince them to take him?" she persists.

"I'm going to stretch the truth a little bit."

She looks at me askance as her index and middle fingers carve a pair of scare quotes into the air above her head.

"Stretch the truth a little bit?"

"Okay, I'm going to lie."

Switchboard puts the call through.

"Hi, this is Luba at the Pink Elephant Detox Centre speaking. How may I help you?"

"Hi Luba, this is Dr. Gray calling from the ER. I have a patient here I'd like to transfer to your facility."

"Certainly. What's your client's name?"

"Rocky Emesis."

"Rocky Emesis?"

"Er, yes. Are you familiar with him?"

"Extremely. When was his last drink?"

"Um . . . I don't think he's had anything so far today."

"What condition is he in right now?"

"Not too bad."

"Would you mind holding for a minute, doctor?"

"No problem."

The instant I'm put on hold, some god-awful Perry Como-esque lounge lizard tune starts playing. Whoever invented muzak should be drawn and quartered. My mind drifts. Luba must be discussing the case with someone higher up the food chain. Does that mean she suspects I'm bullshitting her? I cross my fingers and continue holding.

Nearly a minute later she clicks back on.

"I'd like to speak to the client, please," she says.

Oh crap. Is the Rock Man coherent enough to pass a detox phone screen?

"Um, I think he's in the bathroom right now."

Pretty lame, but it's the best I can do on the spur of the moment.

"He's not vomiting, is he? We definitely do not accept clients who are actively vomiting."

How about if they're passively vomiting?

"Oh no, he's not vomiting, he's just having a pee."

"So he'll be out shortly, then. I'll wait for him."

I jog over to Rocky's stretcher. He's fast asleep.

"Rocky! Wake up!"

"Eh?"

"I'm trying to get you a bed at the Pink Elephant. Come talk to the nice lady and tell her you're okay."

"Feel kinda pukey."

"Just tell her you feel all right!"

"Okay, okay."

I drag him over to the phone.

"Hi, Luba. This is Dr. Gray again. Here's Rocky."

I hand Rocky the phone. Is it just my imagination, or does he look a little green? Must be the fluorescent lights.

"Hello?" I hear Luba say.

"Huurr...."

"Hello?"

"Huuurrrraaaalp!" replies Rocky as he covers the telephone with more Pop Tarts and Big Macs.

I guess I'll be admitting him after all!

Alanna's Birth

On the evening of June 2, 1993, Jan went into labour. The next morning our eldest daughter, Ellen, was born. Everything went smoothly.

On September 3, 1994, our second daughter, Kristen, arrived. Once again there were no complications.

By mid-October the following year Jan was two weeks away from the end of her third pregnancy. Over the preceding two weeks she had noticed a slight reduction in fetal movements, but it hadn't been enough of a decline to concern us. On the morning of October 21 the baby stopped moving altogether. We contacted Miles, our family doctor. He was partway through a 24-hour shift in the emergency department. He asked Jan to come in for a non-stress test. To our relief, during the test the baby stirred a little. There wasn't much beat-to-beat variability, though, so Jan was admitted for induction of labour.

By suppertime the Syntocinon drip was producing regular contractions and active cervical dilatation. At about 7:00 p.m. we started to see a few late decelerations. They made me jittery. I don't do obstetrics, but I know late decelerations can sometimes be a sign of fetal distress. Half an hour later an artificial rupture of membranes was performed. The amniotic fluid that gushed out was nearly black with meconium. Our baby was in trouble.

Switchboard was asked to put the OR team on alert. As Miles deliberated over whether or not to proceed directly to a C-section, one of the ward nurses rushed into the room to show him a rhythm strip from an inpatient who was complaining of feeling light-headed. His heart rate was only 30, and his blood pressure was 75 systolic. Miles and I looked at the tracing together and concluded he was in complete heart block.

I knew exactly what he was thinking: *This can't wait.* Now he had a second critically ill patient to deal with, and we were the only two doctors in the building. On the monitor behind Miles I could see our baby's heart rate was taking an extraordinarily long time to recover from the last uterine contraction. I caught Jan's eye. She looked scared.

"How about if you take care of Jan and the baby and I'll go treat this guy in heart block?" I offered.

"Good idea," he said. He turned his attention back to the fetal heart monitor. I abandoned my wife and followed the nurse back to the cardiac patient's room.

First we started him on a dopamine drip and titrated it up until his pulse and blood pressure improved. We then attached the external pacemaker to his chest and tested it to make sure it would work properly if we needed it in a hurry. Once that was finished I got on the horn to the internist on call at the Timmins and District Hospital, which was our closest referral centre. He agreed to insert a transvenous pacer as soon as we got the patient down to their ICU. I called our ambulance attendants and asked them to start working on transfer arrangements. When I hung up the phone and turned around, Miles was standing in the doorway. The look on his face said *bad news*. He gave it to me straight: "The baby's heart rate dropped down to 60 and stayed there. I've scrambled the OR team and we're setting up for an emergency section." My guts went ice cold.

I went into the operating room to spend a few minutes with Jan before the surgery. My colleagues were bustling about setting up equipment, but the only thing I could hear was the *beep . . . beep . . . beep . . .* of the fetal heart monitor. It was agonizingly slow.

Our regular anaesthetist was out of town that day, but fortunately for us a retired GP-anaesthetist in the community bravely volunteered to put Jan under. When he was ready to begin the induction, Trish the charge nurse shooed me out of the room.

"Go on now. Today you're a dad, not a doctor. I'll call you when we're done." It felt strange leaving the OR and hearing the sliding doors snap shut behind me.

This I learned later: Dr. Hill quickly cut through the layers of tissue until he got to the uterus. He opened it up, reached in and began to pull. Several seconds passed and still no head emerged. He kept working at it. Nothing.

"What's wrong?" someone asked.

"Stuck."

He continued struggling. Sweat beaded on his brow. Eventually he muscled the head out. It was purple. The baby's eyes were closed. She wasn't breathing.

"Cord's around the neck. Damned tight," he muttered.

He strained until he was able to pry the noose-like cord encircling her neck and wriggle it over her head. She remained limp and unresponsive.

"Another loop," he said as he removed a second strangulating coil of umbilical cord from her neck. "And another. And *another!*"

The cord had been wrapped around her neck four times, choking her every time she tried to move. He hauled the rest of her flaccid body out of the uterus and cut the cord.

Miles grabbed the Ambu bag and started ventilating her. While he bagged, Catherine, a nurse who often helped with neonatal resuscitations, listened for a heartbeat. It was barely detectable. She immediately began chest compressions. They worked together feverishly. Moments later the Ambu bag shattered into half a dozen pieces. Catherine and Miles stared at each other, wide eyed. This was unprecedented. The equipment is tested regularly.

"We need another Ambu bag, *stat!*" Miles yelled at Trish.

"That's the only one for newborns we have in the OR! I'll go get one from the delivery room on unit 4!" She darted out of the room. Our child lay inert on the table. Catherine started mouth-to-mouth resuscitation. Miles took over chest compressions.

I was standing in the hallway just outside the OR when Trish burst through the sliding doors. Arms and legs flailing, she looked like the devil himself was chasing her. When she saw me she stopped running, said "Hi" nervously, and speed-walked over to the door to unit 4. She went in and shut the door quietly behind her. The instant it closed I could hear her sprinting down the hallway. I leaned against the wall and tried to breathe. I didn't know what to do. Should I go inside and try to help? Would I be able to make any sort of meaningful contribution, or would I just get in the way?

Trish came thundering back. As soon as she came through the door she glanced at me furtively and slowed to a walk. She was carrying a neonatal Ambu bag. I wanted to scream, "For God's sake, Trish, run!" When she disappeared through the operating room's opaque sliding doors she started running again.

Roughly 20 minutes later Miles came out to see me. He looked grim. I steeled myself for the news that our child was dead.

"It's a girl," he said. "The cord was wrapped around her neck four times and she came out flat. Her one-minute Apgar was only one. We ventilated her and did chest compressions . . ."

. . . but she didn't make it . . .

". . . and she recovered."

"What?" I couldn't hear anything over the blood pounding in my ears.

"She's okay, Donovan, at least for the time being." He smiled.

"Oh, God. Thank you, Miles."

"I'm going to transfer her to Timmins because I'm concerned she may develop delayed respiratory problems."

"Okay."

I went into the OR to meet my new daughter. She had beautiful brown eyes and a shock of curly, black hair. Aside from her rapid respiratory rate she looked remarkably well, considering what she had just been through. Catherine and Trish let me hold her for a little while. I wanted to talk to Jan, but she was still deeply anaesthetized. I asked Trish to tell her I'd call at the first possible opportunity. After that I raced back to our house, sent the babysitter home and arranged to have a neighbour stay with Ellen and Kristen until Jan's parents could fly in from Winnipeg. Once all of that was done I packed an overnight bag and began the long drive down highways 11 and 655 to Timmins.

I arrived at the Timmins and District Hospital to find our EMTs unloading the patient with heart block from the ambulance. He and my daughter had travelled together in the same rig. The attendants informed me they had already taken my daughter to the neonatal unit. When I got there a pediatrician named Dr. Inman was examining her. Her breathing appeared to be more laboured than it had been earlier, but it was hard for me to be sure – it's difficult to maintain any semblance of objectivity when the patient in question is your own child. When he completed his evaluation he told me she was stable for the time being, but that he intended to keep a close eye on her over the next several hours. He felt that due to the asphyxia and meconium it was possible her respiratory status could worsen, and if that occurred she might require intubation. The word *intubation* made me wince – I had visions of barotrauma, collapsed lungs, chest tubes, chronic pulmonary disease . . . . He patted my shoulder.

"Try not to worry," he said. "She looks like a fighter. I think she'll do all right."

I had planned to rent a room at a nearby hotel, but the pediatrics staff kindly arranged for me to use one of the hospital on-call rooms. I telephoned Jan to let her know what was happening. She described how awful it had been waking up after the C-section to find the baby and me both gone. I tried to reassure her and promised I'd call back soon. After that I went to bed. It took a long time for me to fall asleep. A few minutes later the telephone rang. It was Dr. Inman.

"You'd better come back to the unit. Your daughter's getting worse. I think we're going to have to intubate her."

"I'll be right there."

I hung up the phone and cried.

She looked ghastly. Her respiratory rate was well over 70, and her chest and abdomen heaved with each breath. Despite maximal supplemental oxygen her blood oxygen saturations (sats) were only in the low 80s. Dr. Inman explained that although it still wasn't clear whether the problem was transient tachypnea of the newborn, respiratory distress syndrome or meconium aspiration, if she wasn't put on a ventilator soon she'd tire out and stop breathing. I gave my consent for the procedure and left the room.

I wanted to stay with her, but I couldn't bear to witness my own child being intubated.

When I returned the tube was in place and a respiratory therapist was bagging her. Her oxygen sats had climbed to 90 percent and her colour was better.

"The procedure went well," Dr. Inman said. "Right now she's heavily sedated. You'd better go get some sleep. You have a long day ahead of you tomorrow – we'll be flying her down to the neonatal ICU at McMaster first thing in the morning."

The Medevac jet arrived at 10:00 a.m. The transfer team consisted of two NICU nurses. Like everyone else who had treated our daughter (now named Alanna) thus far, they were real pros – meticulous, skillful, and caring. They reviewed the entire case, examined her thoroughly, started two more IVs and switched her over to their own infusion pumps. After communicating with their base neonatologist they adjusted some of her medications. They then detached her from the hospital ventilator, put her in their specialized transfer isolette and reconnected her to a portable ventilator. Once all that was finished they pulled out a Polaroid camera, snapped a picture of her and handed it to me. I thanked them and put it in my knapsack. I later found out that in cases where critically ill infants die shortly after Medevac, oftentimes the pre-transfer snapshot is the only photograph the parents have of their baby taken while the child was alive. I asked the team how I'd find McMaster Children's Hospital when I got to Hamilton. They said as long as there were no other patients requiring air ambulance evacuation they'd make room for me on the jet. I could hardly express my gratitude. An hour later we were in the air.

A ground ambulance met us at the airport in Hamilton and drove us to the hospital. Alanna had held her own during the transfer. It was beginning to look like she might survive this ordeal. As we navigated the hospital corridors on our way to the NICU, thoughts I had been keeping tightly caged broke free: Did she go too long without oxygen? Was she brain-damaged? Would she develop cerebral palsy or be profoundly handicapped? The uncertainty was maddening.

The NICU was a brightly lit sea of chaos. Each isolette was like a life raft bobbing in the turbulence. Some of the infants within the isolettes weren't much bigger than the palm of my hand. It was hard not to stare. I tried to stay out of the way as the transfer team got Alanna settled in. Once the changeover was complete I had a brief meeting with the attending neonatologist. He said he planned to keep Alanna on her existing ventilator settings for the rest of the day. If she remained stable, they would start trying to wean her off in the morning. He asked me where I'd be staying in Hamilton. I had no clue. He gave me the address and phone number of a nearby Ronald McDonald house. I called them and secured a room. I then pulled up a seat and spent the rest of the day watching my daughter's fragile little chest rise and fall in synch with the mechanical bellows.

To everyone's surprise, Alanna tolerated weaning exceptionally well. After two days of ventilatory support she graduated to breathing on her own. Shortly after she was liberated from the ventilator her nurse wrapped her in a warm blanket and let her sit with me in a rocking chair. It was wonderful. I wanted to cradle her in my arms forever.

That afternoon I asked the neonatologist if he had any idea how she was doing cognitively. He said it was difficult to predict such things this early in the recovery phase, but that NICU infants who were able to breastfeed successfully had a significantly higher likelihood of being neurologically intact. He recommended Jan be brought to Hamilton to bond with Alanna and initiate breastfeeding. I spoke to Miles about it. He worked some phone magic, and two days later Jan was admitted to one of McMaster's postpartum wards.

The ink hadn't yet dried on my wife's admission papers before we were on our way to the NICU. Alanna's nurses knew Jan was coming and that she'd be trying to breastfeed, so there was hint of excitement in our little corner of the room. Jan and I were both nervous. The words of the neonatologist weighed heavily on our minds: *NICU infants who were able to breastfeed successfully had a significantly higher likelihood of being neurologically intact.* Jan picked up Alanna and hugged her for several minutes. It was their first encounter.

When we felt we were ready, a nurse led us to an adjacent room and closed the door so we could have some privacy. Jan sat in a chair, slid part of her hospital gown to the side and undid one of the flaps of her nursing bra. She then put our daughter to her breast.

Alanna rooted around aimlessly for what seemed like an awfully long time. Our hearts sank. We put her mouth closer to its target. She fussed and fidgeted a while longer, then suddenly latched on and began gulping milk down at a furious pace. When the breast was completely drained she fell asleep, content. Jan and I were delirious with joy. Our baby was going to be fine.

Alanna hit all her milestones early. She's a crackling ball of energy who enjoys gymnastics, trampoline, volleyball, piano, art and reading. She has never exhibited any ill effects related to her traumatic birth. We consider ourselves to be extremely lucky.

Snip, Snip

When I was single I always said I wanted to have eight kids. Eight kids! Can you imagine? I got a serious reality check when our first child was born. Ellen was a wonderful baby, but caring for her was a lot more work than I had anticipated. Feeding, burping, bathing, changing, rocking, walking, entertaining – it was a full-time job.

Kristen arrived 15 months after Ellen. She was equally marvellous, but following her birth our workload seemed to triple rather than double.

Alanna made her dramatic debut 13 months later. Suddenly we were up to our eyeballs in dirty diapers. Jan started using the word "vasectomy" a lot. Naturally, I pretended not to hear her.

One frisky night about two months after Alanna's birth, Jan and I forgot to take appropriate precautions. The next morning I went to my office and returned with the morning-after pill. The first dose left her feeling queasy, so that evening when it was time for the final set of pills Jan considered not taking them. She telephoned her mother in Manitoba for her opinion on the matter. My usually demure mother-in-law mulled it over for about one-tenth of a second before hollering: "For God's sake, Janet, take the pills!"

Jan took them. The next day I visited Miles and requested a vasectomy.

When you're an MD in a small hospital it sometimes feels weird shedding your lab coat and morphing from doctor into patient, but what's the sense of driving hundreds of kilometres to undergo procedures that can very capably be performed by your own colleagues? On V-Day I arrived at the hospital bright and early. After registering at the front desk I went to the patients' locker room and changed into one of those ridiculous Barbie-sized gowns that always leave half your backside exposed. Who designs those things, anyway? As I walked to the operating room, a trio of ER nurses I work with passed me in the hallway.

"Snip, snip," they cackled.

"Yeah, I love you guys, too. Say hi to Macbeth for me!" I stepped through the sliding doors and into the OR.

Irene the head OR nurse was a cheerful, matronly type.

"Dr. Gray, I see you're here to get 'fixed' this morning! Har-har! Come, lie down!" She patted one of the operating room tables. I reclined on the cold table and tried to relax, but it's hard to unwind when you're minutes away from having the family jewels carved up. After Irene finished setting up the surgical accoutrements, Dr. Hill arrived. The quintessential man of few words, he pulled on his gloves and padded over to me.

"Ready?"

"I guess."

Irene lifted up the front of my gown to expose "the field." The room was chilly, and as a result "the field" had shrunken considerably. Fortunately for my self-esteem, there were no gales of hysterical laughter. After scrubbing the area with antiseptic solution, Dr. Hill picked up a syringe.

"Freezing," he said. The injection wasn't nearly as painful as I had expected, but I broke into a sweat nonetheless.

"It's all right, Dr. Gray," said Irene. "Here's a cool cloth for your forehead." The cloth was surprisingly soothing. I closed my eyes and felt my body begin to loosen. A few seconds later Dr. Hill began cutting.

I daydreamed.

Hey, this isn't so bad . . . .

"Gauze," said Dr. Hill.

My afternoon office is pretty reasonable today, so with any luck I should be home by 4:30 . . . .

"Forceps," said Dr. Hill.

That'll work out well, because we have a 5:00 appointment for a family portrait at the photo studio.

"Sponge," said Dr. Hill.

As long as I don't have to lift the kids, I'll be fine . . . .

"Cautery," said Dr. Hill.

What'd he say? Cautery? Down there?

Zzzzt! Zzzzt! ZZZZZZZZZZZT!

The world's biggest lightning bolt crashed into an exquisitely sensitive part of my anatomy. I arched so rigidly, only my heels and the back of my head remained in contact with the table.

"Yaaaaaaaaugh!"

Dr. Hill looked sideways at me.

"Did you feel that?"

"YES!"

"Oh. Sorry. Irene, could you get me some more freezing please?"

Even though the rest of the procedure was completely painless, I was so paranoid about the possibility of another close encounter with Thor that I wasn't able to relax. When everything was finished I thanked Dr. Hill and Irene and gimped back to the locker room.

Due to a few last-minute add-ins, my office didn't finish until 5:00. I raced home to get ready for the portrait. While I changed into fresh clothes Jan asked me if I was sore.

"It throbs like hell," I replied. "I'll take some Tylenol when we get back." We rounded up the kids and drove to the studio.

"Okay Janet, move Ellen a little bit closer to you. Donovan, could you please lift up Kristen and Alanna and put them on your lap?"

"But –"

"Trust me, it'll make a great shot."

"But –"

"I'm telling you, it'll be perfect. That's right . . . now Alanna . . . good. Um, Donovan?"

"Yes?"

"Are you okay? You look like you just got kicked in the you-know-whats . . . ."

Last Call

Recently I was paged to the emergency department at 3:00 a.m. to stitch up another Jethro. This guy was totally hammered. The story was that he was drinking peacefully with his honey when all of a sudden she up and smashed him in the head with a beer bottle. Damn! Second time she's done that this month! Funny how these guys fall prey to so many unprovoked attacks. I've had several drinks with my wife over the years, and I honestly can't remember her ever bashing my head in with a beer bottle.

Anyway, I set up all of my suturing material, cleaned off his shard-filled forehead and was just about to begin stitching when he yammered, "Hey! W-w-w-wait a minute!"

"Why?"

"I gotta take a leak."

He rolled off the stretcher, staggered to the adjoining bathroom and slammed the door shut. Moments later I was treated to the sound of a torrential stream of used beer. Within a minute he was finished.

Watching him navigate his way back to the stretcher brought to mind images of a sailor trying to walk across a ship's deck in the middle of a typhoon. He plopped back down on the gurney and promptly fell asleep. It wasn't long before he was snoring like a hippo.

I quickly sewed him up (no need for local anaesthetic *this* time, folks), peeled off my gloves and got up to make arrangements for him to be observed in the department for a few hours.

I was halfway out the door when I heard a slurry, nearly unintelligible, "Heyyy doc, hang on a shehcond . . . come ovah here . . . ."

I turned back, intrigued. Was this guy actually going to thank me?

That's a rarity at 3:00 a.m. Most times I consider myself lucky if I don't get barfed on.

"Heyyy doc . . . ."

"Yes?"

"Can you lend me 20 bucks?"

Drug Charades!

Anyone who's worked in an ER knows about drug seekers. They're those incredibly annoying chuckleheads who are forever trying to con us into giving them prescriptions for certain drugs. OxyContin is their Holy Grail, but Percocet, Dilaudid, fentanyl patches, or just about any narcotic will do. Sedatives and stimulants are also welcomed with open arms.

Drug seekers all seem to have cribbed notes from the same manual. They come to the ER after regular clinic hours because they know it's harder for us to crosscheck their hinky stories when other doctors can't be reached. It's not uncommon to hear tales of woe involving pills that have been misplaced, stolen or eaten by the family pet. To improve their odds of getting something high on their wish list they usually claim to be either allergic or immune to all non-narcotic analgesics.

Most of these characters hobble to their allotted cubicle so melodramatically, you'd think they were on the brink of death. They're quick to display any old wounds or surgical scars they might have. Those with no physical evidence of disease to bolster their credibility usually complain of disorders that are difficult to quantify objectively such as headache or back pain. Most seasoned ER docs come to automatically suspect malingering whenever unknown patients present with symptoms of this ilk. This attitude is unfortunate, because it undoubtedly causes us to treat some bona fide sufferers with less compassion than they deserve.

Some of the more inventive drug seekers can really put on a good show. A few years ago one fellow suckered me into giving him intravenous morphine for presumed kidney stones several times until

I clued in to the fact that he only writhed about in agony when he had an audience. When I tiptoed back to his room and observed him surreptitiously he was humming a Def Leppard tune while leafing through an old *People* magazine. As it turned out, he had been covertly adding blood to his urine samples to trick me into thinking he had hematuria. Why on earth would someone with that much drive and creativity waste his time slumming in my ER? He should be down in Hollywood making millions alongside DiCaprio and Depp.

The list of popular swindles and scams is as long as your arm, but an exhaustive review of them all is not what I had in mind for today. No, today I just want to talk about a small subgroup of highly entertaining drug seekers: the Charaders.

In regular charades one player pantomimes a role or phrase while the others try to guess what it is. A correct guess results in jubilation and a strong feeling of camaraderie. In Drug Charades, the patient ropes the unwitting doctor into a game of trying to guess the name of the medication they're after. Although they don't mind dropping Godzilla-sized clues to facilitate the process, they usually try not to say the actual name of the drug themselves. Why? They're hoping the fleeting euphoria the physician experiences when he or she finally guesses correctly will help generate a big, fat prescription.

A game of Drug Charades involving a novice physician and a veteran drug seeker might go something like this:

"Good evening, sir! I'm Floogie Howser, Doogie's younger brother. How can I help you?"

"Well, this morning I accidentally dropped my pills into my neighbour's aquarium and his guppies ate them all."

"My goodness! Are they okay?"

"What?"

"The fish! Are they okay?"

"Oh, yeah, they're fine; just a little sleepy. Listen, is there any way you could refill the prescription for me? I'm not supposed to go without my pills, and my regular doc's on vacation in Antarctica."

"No problem, sir! What kind of pills were they?"

"Painkillers."

"Do you remember the name?"

"Not really, doc – I don't pay much attention to that sort of thing. I think it started with a P, if that's any help."

"P?"

"Yes."

"Gee, I can't recall the names of any painkillers that start with the letter P."

"P-e-r, I think it was."

"P-e-r?"

"Yes."

"Per, per . . . I'm awfully sorry, but I'm drawing a complete blank."

"Per-co-something. They were round and white."

"Per-co, round and white, Per-co . . . Hey! Could it have been Percocet?"

"That's it! Wow, doc, you're incredible!"

"Thanks!"

"So . . . can I get some?"

"Certainly! Will 200 be enough?"

Once in a while I like to have a little fun with Charaders:

"Hi, Mr. Pinkman, my name is Dr. Gray. How can I help you today?"

"Well, doc, last night someone broke into my lab, ah, I mean apartment and stole all my pills. Do you think I could get a prescription for some more?"

"Well . . . ."

"Just enough to tide me over until my regular doc gets back."

"What type of pills were they?"

"Painkillers."

"Hmm. Do you remember the name of the medication?"

"I'm not sure, but they were round and white."

"Aspirin?"

"I think the name started with an O."

"O?"

"Yes."

"Orudis?"

"No, that's not it."

"Hmm . . . ."

"It might have been Oxy-Something."

"Oxygen?"
"No."
"Oxymoron?"
"No! Come to think of it, the last three letters were t-i-n."
"Oxytin?"
"Nine letters . . . ."
"OxyBontin?"
"There's a C in it . . . ."
"OxyContin?"
"Yes!"
"Never heard of it."

Haute Cuisine

A few weekends ago Jan and I were scheduled to return to Hogtown to try our luck at another show and fancy restaurant, but our flight got snowed out. Undaunted, we decided to give one of our little town's newer eateries a try. After securing a babysitter we donned our finest and headed out.

The moment we entered we knew it wasn't going to be a five-star culinary experience. For starters, the oversized television set above the bar was broadcasting a WWF wrestling match at teeth-rattling volume. Some steroidal goon in a lucha libre mask and a velvet cape was whacking a similarly attired Cro-Mag over the head with a metal folding chair. The other immediately obvious problem was that there were only five people in the entire restaurant – a group of four chatty snowmobilers plus a waitress who didn't look much older than the babysitter we had just left behind at our house. So much for ambiance.

Our waitress led us past dozens of empty tables only to stop at one right beside the garrulous quartet. The stench of gasoline was overpowering.

"Is this table okay?" she asked.

"How about somewhere a little more, uh, private?" I replied, *sotto voce*. She moved us to a more suitable spot, gave us our menus and departed.

Five minutes later she returned to take our drink orders. Jan requested something a friend had told her the restaurant stocked – Heisenberg on tap. The waitress apologetically informed her that it was no longer available because the owner had taken the draft tank over to his other restaurant. Shucks. Jan settled for a Blue Light. I ordered a Sling. Yes, you read that right – a Sling. I love girly drinks, especially the ones with those colourful little umbrellas in them. What can I say?

Our waitress returned with Jan's beer, but no Sling. Turning to me she asked: "Is a Sling the same thing as a Singapore Sling?"

"Yes, it is."

She pulled one of those red bartender drink-mixing books out of her hip pocket, rifled through it and said, "According to this, Singapore Slings are usually made with two ounces of lemon juice." I nodded sagely. "My book also mentions an alternative recipe that calls for two ounces of lime juice instead of lemon juice," she continued. "Which would you prefer?"

"Lemon juice, please," I replied.

She skittered off.

Before long she was back with two tall, yellow drinks on her tray. Neither looked even remotely like any Sling I had ever seen before.

"I made one with lemon juice and the other with lime juice," she beamed. "Check and see which you like best."

I took a sip from the first one. It was incredibly sour.

"I don't think you added enough grenadine," I theorized.

"Grenadine? Darn it! Are these things supposed to have *grenadine* in them?" She consulted her little red bible. "You're right, they *are* supposed to have grenadine! Hang on, I'll be right back!"

She zipped away.

Seconds later she returned with a bottle of grenadine.

"Okay," said our teenybopper waitress. "I'll pour, and you tell me when to quit."

I glanced at Jan. She grinned and took a swig of her Blue Light.

"Go for it," I said.

After a couple of *glubs* I held up my hand and she stopped pouring. We all stared at the one-inch layer of grenadine congealing at the bottom of the glass. My drink was beginning to look like a science experiment gone bad. Our waitress picked up my soup spoon and used it to stir the dubious concoction.

"How does it taste now?" she asked eagerly.

I took a sip. *Yecch!*

"Wonderful!" I said. "Thank you very much."

She heaved a sigh of relief, gathered up her stuff and left.

"Our special this evening is liver and onions."

Liver and onions? Yecch!

"Do you have any fish dishes?" I asked.

"We have some really awesome pickerel, sir."

"Is it bony?"

"I don't think so."

"Okay, I'll give it a try, then."

Jan deliberated for a minute before selecting Weiner schnitzel and noodles with a side order of fresh vegetables. As we waited for our food, she drained the last of her Blue Light. I stirred my vile Sling morosely.

Our food arrived. Jan was disappointed to find her "fresh vegetables" were in fact canned peas. To add insult to injury, when she began eating she discovered the noodles tasted like those lumps that used to form in Cream of Wheat.

"I didn't mind the lumps in Cream of Wheat, but they're not supposed to masquerade as German noodles!" she complained. I snickered. Revenge is so sweet.

"Should have ordered the pickerel," I said smugly. "Brain food, you know."

I cut off a piece and bit into it.

"Ack!"

"What's wrong?" asked Jan.

"Bones!" I gasped. A dense cluster of bones trying its damnedest to assassinate me, to be precise. I gingerly extracted the razor-like spicules one by one. Subsequent mouthfuls weren't any better. After several attempts I gave up and turned my attention to the accompanying rice and broccoli. Both were insipid.

At the end of the meal, our food was virtually untouched. When our waitress returned she looked worried.

"Was everything okay?" she asked.

"Splendid. Do you have any decaf?"

"All we have is Sanka," she said.

The only thing worse than no coffee is Sanka. I'd sooner drink bilge water.

"Um, maybe we'll just take the check now," I replied.

We left her a big tip. I'm guessing she used it to purchase the new Backstreet Boys album. Or perhaps a couple of tubes of Clearasil. Small town living. There's no life like it!

"I swear, he wasn't breathing!"

The other day I was working in the ER when suddenly the overhead PA system crackled to life: "Code Blue in the Special Care Unit, Code Blue!"

I abandoned my patient in mid-sentence and belted out of the department. As I passed the operating room I was joined by both our surgeon and our anaesthetist.

At the entrance to unit 4 we nearly collided with four ambulance attendants on their way to assist at the code. The seven of us thundered down the hall like a herd of stampeding rhinos.

We came crashing into the room only to find that two other doctors, a medical student, a respiratory therapist and at least half a dozen nurses had already beaten us to the punch. It was standing room only.

I wormed my way to the bedside to see how the resuscitation was progressing. To my surprise, the patient was sitting bolt upright in his bed. His eyes were as wide as saucers. He was looking fearfully at the medical student, who happened to be brandishing the defibrillator paddles. There was a nursing student with Ferrari-red cheeks at the foot of the bed.

"I swear, he wasn't breathing!" she was telling anyone who'd listen. After a fair bit of grumbling the mob slowly began to disperse.

As we left the room I heard the anaesthetist mutter, "Code Blue? More like a Code Blue Light!"

Rollover Rob *(The Adamantium Man)*

Last Wednesday night the ER was flat-out ridiculous. Think TARFU. No, scratch that. More like DEFCON 1. I didn't get home until well after two in the morning. I shed my clothing and fell asleep within seconds. Five minutes later the phone rang. It's uncanny how often that happens.

"A-roo?" I groaned into the receiver. *Wait a minute, that's not English.* "Hello?"

"Hi Dr. Gray. Sorry to wake you, but I've got an intoxicated 24-year-old man who was just in a rollover. He has a swollen left elbow, some contusions and several superficial lacerations."

"Coupla minutes."

As I fumbled around in the dark in search of my discarded scrubs I recited my well-worn motivational mantra: *I love my job, I love my job, I love my job* . . . .

When I got to the hospital I hung up my jacket and went to the ER. I must have looked even more pathetic than usual because the nurse supervisor apologized again for waking me up.

"It's okay," I said. "Where is he?"

She pointed to room F.

A tattoo-laden critter in a Kid Rock T-shirt, muddy black jeans and roach-killer cowboy boots was sprawled on the stretcher. He stank of booze. When he saw me he grinned widely and yelled, "HEY, BUDDY!"

"I'm not your buddy," I growled. He looked surprised. I guess back on his home planet everyone's cheerful at 2:45 a.m. "What's your name?"

"Rob."

"Okay Rob, take off everything except your underwear."

Just then a teenage girl wearing more makeup than your average circus clown barged in and addressed my new patient.

"Hey, baby, your lighter's not working," she said. "Got any matches?"

"Who are you?" I asked.

"Rob's girlfriend."
"Were you in the accident?"
"Nope."
I jerked my thumb towards the door.
"Out."
Bozette hightailed it out of the room. While I shut the door, Rob stripped down to his Fruit of the Looms.

As I examined him I got more of a history. The saga went something like this: Rob and his merry band of cretins had been drinking heavily all night. Sometime around 1:30 he managed to convince his sidekicks Little Klutz and Friar Schmuck to drive him to a neighbouring town so he could look up his ex-girlfriend and three-month-old son. They were doing an estimated 150 kilometres per hour when their car parted company with the highway. Not surprisingly he didn't recollect too much about the crash itself, but he did remember kicking out the remnants of the rear windshield and crawling away from the smouldering wreckage. In order to avoid the police with all their pesky questions and breathalyzers, the gormless trio fled the scene. When Rob got back to his apartment his current girlfriend took one look at him and dragged him to the ER to get checked out.

Aside from an abundance of minor scrapes and bruises, Rob appeared to be all right. Even his nipple rings were intact. The only thing of concern was his left elbow – it was moderately swollen and he wasn't moving it well. I asked switchboard to call the x-ray tech in. I was feeling a little guilty about the way I had summarily kicked his girlfriend out earlier, so I asked the receptionist to allow her to return so they could sit together while he waited for his films. My conscience appeased, I hunkered down at the main desk in the ER and began my charting.

As soon as his girlfriend arrived they started talking:
"You okay, baby?"
"Yeah, I'm fine."
"What'd the doctor say?"
"I just need a couple of x-rays, no big deal."

"Will you need a cast?"

"Dunno."

"What about one of those shots for, you know, that, like, lockjaw thingy?"

"Naw, I got one of those after I got my tats in jail a coupla years ago."

"Oh, that's good. You sure you're okay, baby? How many times did you roll?"

"Six or seven times, max. Like I said, no big deal. I've been in lots of rollovers before. I just walk away from them."

"Oooh, Robby," she squealed, "you're the best!"

Yep, that's a really important trait to take into account when considering a potential mate – the ability to walk away from rollovers. You just never know when it might come in handy!

Drinking Problem

Several nights ago a 14-month-old boy with a cough was brought to our emergency department. While I obtained the history from his mother, the little fellow happily explored the room. After a couple of minutes he toddled back to her and reached for the half-full cup of Tim Hortons coffee she had been sipping from.

"Eh! Eh!" he grunted.

"Jack-Jack want coffee?" she asked.

"Eh! Eh!" he confirmed.

She handed him the cup. I watched in disbelief as he noisily slurped the rest of the java down. When he was finished he burped loudly, hucked the empty cup on the floor and wobbled away.

"You let your 14-month-old son drink coffee?" I asked incredulously.

"Oh, Jack drinks whatever I drink," was her reply.

* * *

Blood

At 8:30 this morning a trucker accidentally dropped a large hunting knife on his left foot. The blade pierced the skin and embedded itself deep in the bone. When he pulled it out, a miniature geyser of blood erupted. He tried to staunch the flow with some towels, but within a few seconds they were soaked. He drove his rig to our hospital and limped into the ER. The triage nurse applied a tight pressure dressing and had me paged.

By the time I arrived, the minor trauma room was saturated with the odour of blood. It washed over me in waves as I stitched up the wound. Traces of it clung to my clothes long after the patient departed.

Just as the ghostly scent of blood was beginning to fade from my memory, an industrial accident victim was brought in. He had crushed his right hand between two steel plates. Fortunately no bones were broken, but several of his fingernails had blood trapped underneath them. The nail bed hematomas were causing a lot of pain. To relieve his discomfort I drilled holes through the damaged nails with an 18-gauge needle. The smell of the draining blood gave me a weird feeling of déjà vu.

An hour later a drunken 25-year-old who had just put his fist through a plate-glass window staggered up to the receptionist's desk. Arcs of blood sprayed from his jagged wrist laceration in perfect sync with his heartbeat. I hustled him into a treatment room and began suturing. After about a dozen stitches the bleeding reluctantly came under control.

My next patient asked me to look at a mole on her shoulder that had recently enlarged. It was multi-coloured, elevated and irregular. She didn't have a family doctor, so I removed it for her. More molecules of blood escaped into the air.

After the mole excision I went to the dirty utility room to deposit my used scalpel blade and needles. One of my colleagues had just finished a busy lumps-and-bumps clinic, so the sharps disposal container was nearly full. When I opened it I was assaulted by the odour of fresh blood once again.

Our bedroom is bathed in moonlight.
The clock on the wall reads a quarter past midnight.
I'm lying in bed, waiting for the Sandman.

I can still smell blood.

Paralyzed

Tharn – *a fictional word used in the Richard Adams novel* Watership Down *to describe rabbits frozen in terror at the sight of the headlights of an oncoming car.*

One night I was working in the emergency department when the nursing supervisor advised me an ambulance had just been dispatched to pick up a teenager who had collapsed. A few minutes later EMS radioed to notify us they were coming in hot with an unstable cardiac patient.

They rolled in with a drowsy 15-year-old boy named Johnny. He had a pulse of 230 and a dangerously low blood pressure. We got him into a gown, administered oxygen and put him on the cardiac monitor.

He wasn't my patient, but I vaguely remembered seeing him in the ER a few years prior for issues related to an irregular heartbeat. At the time a pediatric cardiologist had strongly recommended Johnny undergo a relatively minor procedure on the electrical pathways of the heart to eradicate the disorder.

"Did you ever get that heart procedure done?" I asked.

"No."

"Why not?"

"I didn't want it."

"Does your heart beat too fast sometimes?"

"Yes."

"What do you do when that happens?"

"I take these." He pulled a bottle of heart pills out of his pocket. "I'm supposed to take one three times a day, but sometimes I forget. If my heart's going too fast I take a few extra. I've been doing that a lot lately."

"Where are your parents right now?"

"I just live with my mother. Why?"

"I'm going to need to speak to her."

"About what?"

The pills he was on can sometimes trigger abnormal heart rhythms if not taken as prescribed. Using layman's terms, I advised him that with the current combination of heart disease, unknown levels of cardiac medication in his bloodstream and unstable vital signs, the quickest and safest solution would be for us to provide intravenous sedation and then use special paddles to electrically convert his heart rhythm back to normal.

"You're not doing that to me," he declared.

I telephoned his mother and asked her to come to the ER right away. When she arrived I reviewed the situation with her and explained why it would be better for us to cardiovert her son now, before things got any worse.

"What does Johnny say?" she asked.

"He doesn't want to do it, but he's too young and scared to make a rational decision."

"If he doesn't want it, he doesn't have to have it."

The best alternative to electrical cardioversion was a medication named procainamide, so I started him on an intravenous infusion of it.

Half an hour later his pulse had decreased to 180, but his blood pressure was still too low and he remained in an abnormal heart rhythm. I telephoned a cardiologist for advice. He agreed the optimal treatment was electrical cardioversion, but felt that given the circumstances we could give a second cardiac medication a try. Two doses of the alternate drug had no discernible effect on Johnny's rapid heart rate, so I restarted the procainamide.

By midnight his pulse had declined to 150, but his blood pressure was fading and he was nearly comatose.

I told his mother if we waited any longer to perform the procedure, he would probably die. She consented resignedly. My colleague Serge sedated him and I performed a synchronized cardioversion at 50 joules. His rhythm remained unchanged. I increased the power to

100 joules and shocked him again.

Johnny's heart stopped beating. Stone-cold asystole.

"No pulse!" the emerg nurse shouted.

Time stood perfectly still. The silence was deafening. My body locked up. My brain turned to mush. I couldn't think. I could barely breathe. Serge and I stared at each other blankly. We hadn't anticipated this outcome, and as a result we weren't mentally prepared for it.

Serge's lips twitched spasmodically as he tried to decide what to do next. Finally he said: "Electricity got him into this and it'll get him out of it. Shock him again."

I looked stupidly at the paddles in my hands. The urge to do *something* was overwhelming. From the deepest recesses of my frozen mind a thought struggled to rise. I waited for it. Finally it burst to the surface: *You don't shock asystole!*

"No," I said numbly.

"Okay," he said. "Put the paddles down, then."

I think I was making him nervous. I woodenly returned the paddles to their slots in the defibrillator and watched in a haze as Serge strained to think us through this mess. He was as rattled as I was, but at least he was fighting it.

Suddenly his eyes widened.

"Start CPR!" he shouted. The ambulance attendants sprang into action. "One milligram of epinephrine IV!" He had broken free of his mental gridlock. He grabbed an endotracheal tube and intubated Johnny. Now everyone was moving but me.

The events unfolding around me seemed to be occurring in a surreal, molasses-like slow motion. Although I was fully aware of the fact that I had skillfully dealt with cases worse than this in the past, for some reason I was completely paralyzed. I remained in a near-catatonic state; a fly in amber. I tried to focus on the asystole algorithm, but I simply could not stop thinking, "What did I just do? I've killed this boy." It was awful.

Although my *sang-froid* completely deserted me, fortunately for Johnny my teammates kept their wits about them. They performed excellent chest compressions and lung ventilation. They administered the correct drugs at appropriate intervals. Six inconceivably long minutes later Johnny developed a recognizable cardiac rhythm on the monitor. Seconds later his femoral pulses returned and a blood pressure of 70 systolic was recorded.

By that time my miasma was clearing and I was semi-functional. I ordered a dopamine infusion and got on the phone to the closest ICU with an available bed. Within an hour he was airborne.

Johnny went on to a full recovery and had his cardiac electrical problem fixed a few months later. He has not had any further heart rhythm issues.

As for myself, that night taught me the danger of getting caught flat-footed. I now try to be a good Boy Scout and prepare myself for every eventuality, even though in my heart of hearts I know that there's no way you can be ready for everything all the time. ER workers are, after all, only human.

Rick's Tears

When they told me Rick was coming in by ambulance, I knew right away something was very wrong. Rick never called for EMS, no matter how sick he was. To him, coming in by ambulance was tantamount to admitting defeat. I went to the resuscitation room and started preparing my gear.

Rick was a 35-year-old man who had been waging an intense chess-like battle against cancer for the past five years. Although he wasn't my patient, I knew him fairly well because I had treated him in the ER on several occasions. One thing that always impressed me about him was his relentlessly positive attitude. Rather than walk around in a blue funk bemoaning his fate, he focused his energy on getting better. He had more important things to do than die of cancer. He wanted to spend more time with his wife, Tammy. He planned to help his kids make the awkward transition from childhood to adolescence. He had a business to run and projects to complete. Most cancer victims hope they'll survive. Rick *intended* to.

Death simply wasn't an option.

He demonstrated his indomitable will to live in many ways. When the initial staging tests revealed the cancer was much more widespread than originally expected, his response was, "Well, we'll just have to work a bit harder to get rid of it, that's all." When his first chemotherapy cocktail failed miserably he moved on to the next line of treatment without so much as a backward glance. Plan B was followed by plans C, D, E . . . . One day the cancer disappeared. Extensive testing failed to show any trace of malignancy within his body. Rick was in remission. He was thrilled, but he wasn't surprised – he had fully expected to conquer his foe.

A year later the cancer recurred. At first Rick was despondent, but before long his unflagging optimism returned. Conventional chemotherapy proved to be completely ineffective this time, so he signed up for oncology trials involving experimental drugs. If he was quoted a mere five percent chance of success for a given regimen he'd say, "That's all right – I'm going to be in the lucky five percent." When the drug proved to be a failure he'd shrug and say, "Let's hope the information they got from studying me will help the next guy beat his cancer."

Once in a while a treatment regimen would look promising in the early stages – Rick's tumours would shrink, his blood counts would improve and he'd start to feel better. He would predict with unshakeable confidence that it wouldn't be long before he was rid of his disease. Within a few months, though, the cancer would invariably regroup and resurge, stronger and more resilient than ever. Eventually it became apparent to everyone but Rick that he was not going to win the war.

The attendants hit the door running. "He was awake and talking the whole way here, but when we pulled into the ambulance bay he slumped over and became unresponsive!"

Rick looked sepulchral. He was propped up in the stretcher and leaning heavily to the left. His eyes were vacant and he was barely breathing. I put two fingers to his neck. His carotid pulse was weak. I cupped my hand to his ear and said, "Rick, can you hear me?" He didn't respond. I put my hand in his. "Rick, squeeze my fingers." His hand remained limp. I was reaching for the blood pressure cuff when I noticed his left eye glistening. I stood transfixed as a solitary tear broke free and tracked down his cheek.

A tear from a dying man. *Endgame.* I felt someone walk over my grave. Turning to one of the attendants, I whispered, "What's his code status?"

"I'm not sure, but you can ask his wife – she's right next door in the triage room."

Tammy was distraught. I explained that Rick was moribund and asked if he had ever given any indication as to whether he wanted aggressive interventions in the event his heart stopped beating. She said he had requested no heroic measures be undertaken. We went back to the treatment room together. His blood pressure was hovering around 60 systolic and he was nearly unconscious. It didn't look as though he was going to last long. She held his hand and stroked his thinning hair. The rest of us stood by and waited.

Impossibly, several minutes later he opened his eyes and looked around. He was too weak to talk, but he seemed to recognize Tammy. He obviously wasn't yet ready to relinquish his fragile hold on life. I sequestered his family in the triage room for an impromptu conference and asked if they were in favour of giving him a rapid infusion of intravenous fluids in an attempt to boost his blood pressure. I explained any improvement would likely only be temporary, but that it might give him a few more hours of consciousness. After deliberating for a short time they decided to give it a try.

Halfway through the third litre of saline he arose like Lazarus, asked for a drink of water, and held court with his family. When I asked him what his wishes were regarding end-of-life care, he confirmed he didn't want CPR, defibrillation, intubation or mechanical ventilation. Intravenous fluids were fine, though; he was hoping to keep body and soul together long enough to participate in an exciting new chemo trial scheduled to begin in a couple of weeks.

"You do your job, and I'll do mine," he said to me with a mischievous twinkle in his eye.

Over the course of the next two hours Rick slipped in and out of consciousness. During lucid intervals he would reminisce with his family about happier times. Sometimes he spoke wistfully about up-and-coming treatments he had read about. Not once did he speak of death. Shortly after midnight he lapsed into a coma. I wrote admission orders and transferred him to the medical floor for palliative care. By 3:00 a.m. the emergency department's waiting room was empty. I hung up my lab coat and drove home.

Three hours later my telephone rang. It was a nurse from the medical floor.

"Sorry to wake you, Dr. Gray, but Rick just died."

"I'll be there in a few minutes."

I got out of bed, dressed and returned to the hospital.

Pronouncing someone dead is a strange ritual. It's equal parts medicine, religion and magic. Like falling snowflakes, no two pronouncements are ever the same. Sometimes the body is alone in the room; shrouded in darkness, isolated and abandoned. Other times the room is well lit and packed with family members and friends. Sometimes the dominant mood is sadness. Other times it's relief. No matter how many mourners are present, though, a palpable stillness descends when I enter the room. I become a shaman. My gift is closure.

On this occasion there were seven people clustered around the bed. When I walked in, they all turned towards me expectantly. My fingers gripped the stethoscope in my pocket. For a moment it felt like a string of rosary beads. I approached Tammy and squeezed her shoulder in sympathy.

"Thank you for looking after him earlier," she said.

"You're very welcome," I replied. "I only wish we could have done more. Was he in any pain at the end?"

"No, he looked like he was comfortable."

"Did he ever regain consciousness after he left the emergency department?"

"Yes, a few times. The last time was about half an hour ago. He opened his eyes and spoke to me. I think he must have realized he was about to die."

"What did he say?"

"The fire's gone out."

Rick was recumbent on the bed with his eyes closed. Although it was clear that his life-thread had finally been severed, I could sense the family needed me to confirm it. I lifted his cooling wrist and felt for a radial pulse. There was none. I checked his carotids. Nothing. I placed the diaphragm of my stethoscope directly in front of his bluish lips and listened for breath sounds. Silence. I auscultated his chest for a heartbeat. Once again there was no sign of life. The last thing I usually do is check for a pupillary reflex. I put my right thumb on his left eyelid and gently opened his eye. A solitary tear broke free and tracked down his cheek.

Parenting 101

My next three patients are a young family with mild gastro symptoms. While I obtain a history from the parents their toddler Billy pokes around the room, happy as a clam. I examine the father. I examine the mother. Now it's Billy's turn.

I ask his parents to put him on the stretcher. When his mother leans over to pick him up, Billy goes bonkers. He windmills his arms and screeches, "No!" He then runs behind the stretcher and stares up at us defiantly.

"I don't think he's going to let you look at him," his mother concludes.

"How old is Billy?" I ask.

"He just turned two."

"I think we're in charge here, don't you? Please put him up on the stretcher so I can check him."

She approaches Billy cautiously. He bares his teeth at her like he's some kind of rabid ferret. When she lifts him up, he arches his back, kicks his feet and uncorks a blood-curdling, "No! No! No! NOOOOOO!!!!" Damned if she doesn't put him back down.

"Billy doesn't like doctors," she reiterates.

I'm running out of patience.

"Look, this isn't a democracy – his vote doesn't count. It doesn't really matter if he says no. Just put him on the stretcher anyway."

At this juncture a tiny light bulb appears above her head. *Aha! A brand new concept!* This time she and her husband pick up Billy and deposit him on the stretcher like they mean business.

"Now you sit still, Billy," she says firmly. After putting up a token show of resistance he settles down nicely. I begin my examination.

Adventures in Paralysis *(The Ventilator Blues)*

Every now and then we ER docs supplement our armamentarium with techniques borrowed from other specialties. Rapid sequence intubation (RSI) is one such purloined procedure. It involves using induction and paralytic agents to facilitate emergency endotracheal intubation. In plain English, this means we sometimes give patients who are struggling to breathe drugs that render them comatose and paralyzed. We then move their tongue out of the way with a device called a laryngoscope and quickly advance a hollow 12-inch plastic endotracheal tube (ET tube) past the back of the throat, through the vocal cords and into the trachea (windpipe). When the tube is in place we attach it to an Ambu bag. Squeezing the bag rhythmically results in 100 percent oxygen being delivered to the patient's lungs. Depending on the situation, the ET tube can subsequently be attached to a ventilator.

As the name implies, RSI allows us to rapidly take control of a patient's breathing. Anaesthetists have long used coma-inducing and paralyzing drugs in the OR, but it wasn't until relatively recently that it was recognized there was a role for these medications in the ER as well. RSI is an invaluable adjunct, and it has bailed me out of a number of airway crises. Usually it goes off without a hitch, but once in a while things can get a little hairy. Here are three cases from my *Yikes!* file.

Are You Sure This Stuff Is Going to Help Me Relax?

Several years ago I was working in the ER when we got word an ambulance was on its way in with someone who had been trapped in the basement of a burning building. Before long the paramedics arrived with an uncooperative man in his early 20s. His clothing was badly charred and he was covered in soot. Inspection of his throat revealed a raw, beet-red palate, and his sputum was speckled with carbonaceous material. It was obvious he had suffered significant thermal damage to his upper airway. It is generally recommended that patients with this type of injury be intubated early. If you wait too long, late attempts at securing the airway may prove to be impossible due to massive soft tissue swelling in the throat. In situations where multiple intubation attempts have failed, oftentimes the only remaining airway management option is emergency cricothyroidotomy, i.e., cutting the front of the neck open to directly access the trachea. Rumour has it that incising the neck of a confused, combative burn victim isn't much fun. Intubate early and save yourself a world of grief.

As we stripped off the patient's smouldering clothes and started IVs I advised him of my concerns regarding his airway. When I told him I thought he needed to be intubated he said: "Are you saying you want to stick a tube down my throat and put me on a breathing machine?"

"In a nutshell, yes."

"Yeah, right! Like *that's* ever going to happen! No way, man. I'm out of here." He sat up and pulled out one of his IVs.

"Mr. Cotard, I think you're making a big mistake. Any minute now your throat might begin to swell. If it does, you could suffocate."

"I already told you, there's nothing wrong with me. I'm going home." He started tugging on his remaining IV.

"Hang on," I parried. "What's the big rush? Why don't you stay a little while and let us keep an eye on you? If nothing happens, we'll let you go."

"Okay," he agreed grudgingly. "I'll stay for 10 minutes, max."

With each passing minute he grew more restless and agitated. We had to continually remind him to leave his oxygen mask on. Eventually his oxygen sats began to drop.

"If we wait much longer to intubate you, it may be too late."

"Not a chance!"

Moments later his voice started getting raspy. The ER nurses and I exchanged worried glances. *Vocal cord swelling*. Not long after that he developed stridor, a high-pitched inspiratory wheeze indicative of a precariously narrow upper airway.

"That noise you're making each time you inhale tells us we're running out of time. We have to intubate you now before your airway becomes completely obstructed."

"No way!" he squeaked. "Stay away from me!"

"All right then, at least let me give you something to help you relax a bit."

"Okay."

I drew up four syringes of RSI drugs: thiopental, succinylcholine, pancuronium and diazepam. My patient eyed the syringes suspiciously.

"Are you sure this stuff is going to help me relax?"

"I guarantee it."

I injected the thiopental and succinylcholine into his IV port. Within a minute he was unconscious and paralyzed. I then squeezed a pediatric-sized ET tube through his flambéed vocal cords, hooked him up to a ventilator and shipped him off to the closest burn centre.

We were later advised his inhalation injuries were so severe he required mechanical ventilation for more than a week. His subsequent convalescence was uneventful.

As you can see, occasionally we're forced to override an irrational patient decision in order to save someone from themselves. These situations have the potential to ignite ethical and medicolegal firestorms. Whenever I'm caught in this type of quandary my guiding principle is to do whatever I think is morally imperative and save the worrying about potential repercussions for later. In other words, do the right thing! So far this axiom has not let me down.

How Come She's Not Breathing Anymore?

One night I was paged to the Special Care Unit to evaluate a teenage girl in respiratory distress. The nurse caring for her informed me the patient had presented to the emergency department earlier in the day after having ingested a large quantity of unknown pills. She had been treated with activated charcoal and observed closely in the ER. Nothing untoward had happened, so after a few hours she had been transferred to the unit for further monitoring. Her breathing had started to become laboured a few minutes prior to my being contacted.

The patient's breathing was rapid and shallow. Despite maximal supplemental oxygen, her sats were only 80 percent. Examination, bloodwork and a portable chest x-ray failed to reveal any obvious cause for her abrupt deterioration. I wondered about the possibility of a pulmonary blood clot. Before I could pursue that line of thought any further, her respiratory status took a turn for the worse. I decided to intubate.

I selected my airway tools and calculated the appropriate RSI drug dosages. While the nurse got the medications ready I studied the patient's mouth and neck in an attempt to gauge how difficult it was going to be to intubate her. Her receding chin, small mouth and big tongue all suggested the procedure would be technically challenging. If I paralyzed her and then found myself unable to get the tube in I'd be up the proverbial creek. Like the saying goes, bad breath is better than no breath. I therefore decided to do an awake intubation, meaning I would numb her throat and upper airway with the topical anaesthetic Xylocaine and then gingerly advance the ET tube into place. Once the tube was in, I'd quickly sedate and paralyze her in order to eliminate the possibility of her inadvertently yanking it out. I went over the plan with her in detail. She said she'd try her best to cooperate.

First I flattened her tongue with a tongue depressor and sprayed the back of her throat with Xylocaine. A minute later I instructed her to lie down. I then slid the laryngoscope blade to the back of her throat and sprayed the zone between the posterior throat and the voice box. This caused her to cough and splutter so much I had to withdraw the scope and give her a minute to recover. On the next attempt I was able to get the blade a bit further down, but when I began spraying she reached up and tried to grab my hand. Not good. I removed the scope again.

"Are you okay?" I inquired.

"Yes. Sorry about that – it was just a reflex," she panted.

I turned to the nurse and whispered: "This looks like it'll be a tough intubation. I'm going to want to give her the thiopental and sux to sedate and paralyze her as soon as the tube's in place so she doesn't pull it out."

"Okay, I'll have them both ready."

I went in again. This time I saw a sliver of the epiglottis, which is the lid of the voice box. The vocal cords lie directly beneath it. When I squirted the epiglottis with Xylocaine she started coughing violently. She then began twisting and rolling around on the bed. I withdrew the scope and waited for her to settle. When she calmed down I asked, "Are you okay?" No answer. "Miss Pickwick?" Silence. Something was wack. Was it just my imagination, or did she appear to be unnaturally still?

"Hey, wait a minute – how come she's not *breathing* anymore?"

The nurse checked the patient's IV line and gasped.

"I inserted the loaded syringes of thiopental and succinylcholine into her IV port and left them there so we'd be able to inject as soon as you got the tube in! Both syringes are completely empty – she must have self-injected just now when she rolled over!" *Yikes!*

Her oxygen sats entered free fall. I asked the nurse to apply firm pressure to the patient's cricoid cartilage to reduce her risk of aspirating stomach contents. In the meantime I attempted to ventilate her lungs with the Ambu bag. Even using both hands I couldn't get a good seal with the mask. Her sats hit 70 percent. I put the laryngoscope back down her throat and hunted for her vocal cords. I could barely see the epiglottis, never mind the cords.

"O2 sat 60 percent!" shouted the nurse. A multitude of monitor alarms started beeping simultaneously. I went into Hulk mode and pulled on the laryngoscope so hard, it's a wonder the patient's entire body didn't lift off the bed. Miraculously, her vocal cords popped into view. I vaguely recall my hands trembling a little as I guided the ET tube home.

Miss Pickwick went on to a complete recovery.

Let Me Help You With That, Doctor

A while back I was called to the medical floor to see a patient who was developing pulmonary edema, or fluid on the lungs. Despite aggressive medical therapy and BiPAP she was becoming increasingly short of breath. She needed to be tubed and put on a ventilator. I set out my equipment and assessed her airway. Her anatomy was favourable and there was nothing to suggest she'd be a difficult intubation. The only wrinkle was that if I knocked her out with thiopental, her already-lowish blood pressure could bottom out completely. I elected to sedate her lightly with midazolam, paralyze her with succinylcholine and then slip the endotracheal tube in. Once the tube was in place I'd sedate her more heavily. I explained the game plan to her and she gave me the green light to proceed.

I injected 3 mg of midazolam and 100 mg of succinylcholine into her IV port. Succinylcholine usually effects paralysis within a minute or so. After a minute of cricoid pressure and bagging I put the laryngoscope in her mouth. I could see her vocal cords clearly. My ET tube was on a sterile towel next to the patient's head. I didn't want to lose sight of my target, so I said, "Could somebody please pass me the tube?" The patient picked it up and handed it to me. I almost quailed. "Hey! Aren't you supposed to be paralyzed?" I asked.

"Am I? I guess it didn't work," she mumbled around the laryngoscope blade in her mouth. "Are you almost finished? This is kind of uncomfortable."

I removed the scope and inspected the bottle of succinylcholine. It was nowhere near its expiry date. I checked the patient's IV line. It was patent. *What the hell?*

"Ms. Selwyn, we're going to try that again."

"Okay, doctor."

I gave her a touch more midazolam plus another 150 mg of succinylcholine and waited for her to go limp. Nothing happened.

"Aren't you paralyzed yet?"

"Sorry, no."

I sprayed her throat and upper airway with Xylocaine and tried to do an awake intubation, but when the ET tube reached her vocal cords she started thrashing about. Attempting to pass the tube was like trying to hit a moving target. I was worried about traumatizing her epiglottis and cords, so I pulled the laryngoscope out.

Before I could work out a Plan C, her oxygen sats fell off a cliff. I gave her a ton of midazolam plus a whopping 200 mg of succinylcholine. She still wasn't paralyzed, but at least she was adequately drowsy. When I put the laryngoscope back in her mouth I nearly gagged. It looked as if a tiny grenade had just exploded at the base of her throat. The trauma of the preceding intubation attempt had caused the soft tissues of her upper airway to swell so grotesquely, I couldn't spot anything even remotely recognizable. More and more alarms bleeped as her oxygen sats continued to tank. I was on the verge of asking for the cricothyroidotomy tray and a scalpel when a tiny air bubble appeared on the surface of one of the bruised lumps of flesh at the back of her throat. *That bubble must have just exited the trachea!* I aimed for it and pushed firmly. The tube slid underneath her distorted epiglottis and lodged neatly in the windpipe. *Bingo!*

A few months later I attended an advanced airway management course. One of the instructors informed us that once in a blue moon you run across a bottle of succinylcholine that simply doesn't work. Apparently the anaesthetists call it "Bad Sux." The solution? Toss it out and open a new bottle!

In my next life I'm hoping to come back as a librarian. I can't handle all this excitement!

Koyaanisqatsi (Life Out of Balance)

> *"Things fall apart; the center cannot hold;*
> *Mere anarchy is loosed upon the world . . . ."*
> – William Butler Yeats, *The Second Coming*

Remember that high school science experiment with the tin can? Allow me to refresh your memory. You took a large tin can, sucked all the air out of it with a vacuum pump and then resealed the lid. Within seconds the can caved in, crushed by the surrounding atmospheric pressure. Kids applauded, your science teacher bowed theatrically and the jocks loitering at the back of the class rained an apocalypse of spitballs down on the hapless geeks in the front row. Ladies and gentlemen, I present to you Exhibit A, the Human Tin Can. Watch carefully as the pressure generated by running a busy medical practice while simultaneously attempting to be an involved parent, an attentive spouse and a dutiful son threatens to crush him like a bug. Will he implode? Place your bets, everyone, place your bets!

I, Carnival Duck *(Apologies to I, Claudius)*

I'm on call for our ER every Wednesday night, so I usually take

Thursday mornings off. Or at least, I try to. In theory it makes sense – if I give myself a chance to repay my sleep debt, maybe I'll be able to avoid premature flameout. In reality, though, it doesn't always work out that way. Yesterday was Thursday. Here's how the morning went.

Whether it's my morning off or not, my daughters still have to get to school on time. Accordingly, my alarm clock went off at 6:55 a.m., same as always. I had just gotten home from the hospital about two hours prior, so I spent the next few minutes lurching around the room like an extra from the set of *The Walking Dead*. Eventually I woke up enough to help the girls with their morning rituals. At 8:15 I walked them to the bus stop. A few minutes later I was waving goodbye as their bus pulled away from the curb. I picked up my usual bagel and coffee at Tim Hortons and drove to the hospital. As I ate in the doctor's lounge I formulated a battle plan. I would go directly to the medical floor, see my four inpatients as quickly as possible and then beat a hasty retreat home. I figured if I eliminated all nonessential intra-hospital contact I could be back in bed as early as 9:30. That would give me a solid three hours of sleep before my afternoon office began. The plan sounded good, but was it too optimistic? For doctors, sometimes going from Point A to Point B within a hospital is like running a gauntlet – everyone wants to take a whack at you. Nevertheless, I was determined to succeed. *Avoid all side skirmishes*, I reminded myself as I prepared to exit the lounge.

Beep-beep-beep! I checked my pager's LCD screen. The number for the medical floor flashed at me ominously. *Uh-oh.* I picked up the telephone and called.

"Hi Dr. Gray! Just wanted to let you know two of your patients transferred back from St. Elsewhere last night, so we'll be needing some orders for them."

"Okay."

"You should probably have a look at them, too. One of them keeps dumping his pressure and I think the other one's starting to circle the drain."

So much for getting home by 9:30.

I headed for my locker, which is located a few steps down the hall from the lounge. I hadn't made it a third of the way when the nursing supervisor stopped me.

"There's a problem with that patient of yours who was supposed to go to Timmins for a CT scan of his head today," she declared. "He's a DNR, and the other patient he has to share the ambulance with is a full-code."

She waited for my response. Try as I might, I couldn't determine the point where these two seemingly unrelated lines of data intersected. Eventually I sighed.

"The suspense is killing me."

"According to the new EMS policy, they're not allowed to transport a full-code patient and a no-code patient in the same rig. Two full-codes can share an ambulance, but DNR patients have to be transported by themselves."

"What?"

"New policy."

"Which moron came up with that one?"

"I don't know, but it means they won't be able to take your guy."

"But he already got cancelled once last week due to that blizzard! Besides, he's perfectly stable. Just because he's DNR doesn't mean he's planning on dying anytime soon. He's probably less likely to cash out today than I am."

She smiled wryly and said, "That is exactly what I told the attendants, but they said it didn't matter – rules are rules. Should we rebook him for next week?"

"Don't bother. What's to stop the same thing from happening again next time? Tell you what, let's temporarily switch him to full-code."

"What do you mean?" she asked.

"Discontinue his DNR order and send him in the ambulance with the other guy. When he gets back from his scan I'll reinstate his DNR."

"If central dispatch finds out you're tweaking DNR orders to facilitate transfers, they'll go bananas."

"I've got broad shoulders."

As I was putting on my lab coat one of my colleagues entered the locker room.

"Morning, Donovan! Say, I just noticed that on the new ER schedule you have me on call on the 16th. I won't be able to work that day – my wife's parents are going to be in town."

"You didn't tell me you weren't available to work that day," I whined. Every month I end up revising our call roster six or seven times due to last-minute changes.

"I know, I forgot. Sorry!"

I pulled a copy of the schedule out of my locker.

"Miles is on call the next day. Could you just trade with him?"

"No, that won't work – the outlaws'll be staying the entire weekend."

"Okay, I'll rework things and get back to you."

I sat down with the timetable and brainstormed. Five minutes later I had a viable alternative worked out. *All right, time to get to work!*

I left the locker room and angled across the hallway to our mailboxes. I was glumly eyeing the two new admission cards taped to the front of my box when I heard someone inside the ER mention my name.

". . . I think I just saw him go by. Maybe he stopped at his mailbox."

Oh no. Before I could make like Jimmy Hoffa and disappear, one of the ER nurses stepped out into the hallway and collared me.

"Oh, there you are! I have an outpatient sheet from last night that you forgot to sign."

"Is that all? No problem!" *This'll only take a second!*

I trotted over to the main desk and applied my hieroglyphic scrawl to the sheet.

"Oh, and one more thing," she said. "Remember Mr. Carbuncle? He's the man who had that nasty abscess on his buttock. You lanced it on Monday."

"Yes?"

"He's due to be reassessed this morning to see if his IV antibiotics can be discontinued."

"That's nice."

"He was really hoping you'd be the one to recheck him."

I was on the verge of deferring the task to the doctor on call when Mr. Carbuncle and his wife both leaned out of the doorway of the nearest treatment room and waved at me cheerily.

"Um, sure, I'd be glad to."

When I stepped out of the treatment room, the administrative secretary ambushed me.

"Sorry to bother you, Dr. Gray, but we need to schedule a medical advisory committee meeting. There are a number of pressing items on the agenda that need to be addressed."

"Like what?" *Omigod! Wait! Is it too late for me to retract that question?*

As she summarized the lengthy list I tried my best to nod at appropriate intervals. When I couldn't stand it any longer I interrupted her in mid-sentence.

"How about if we have the meeting next Friday at noon?"

"Next Friday at noon sounds great! I'll send out a memo to everyone." I turned to go. "By the way," she said, "The CEO is going to need your help with the upcoming hospital accreditation. Do you think you'll be able to . . . ."

Administrative duties fulfilled, I made a beeline for the medical ward. As I was passing switchboard the operator waved me over to her desk.

"That specialist you were trying to track down yesterday is returning your call," she said.

"Oh, that's okay – I managed to get the patient I was calling him about stabilized and transferred somewhere else, so I don't need to speak to him anymore."

"You might as well tell him that yourself – he'll be on the line any second now. What number should I put it through to?"

"But – "

"Here he is now. I'll patch it through to the phone right behind you in Medical Records."

Dr. Verbose was in a particularly chatty mood. At his request, we reviewed the details of the case I had been trying to reach him about. He seemed to be satisfied with the way things had turned out. While we were talking I noticed someone from the business office begin to hover nearby. Before long an ER nurse joined her. The instant I hung up they descended like ravens.

"Dr. Gray, the architect wants to know when he'll be able to meet with you to go over the new medical clinic plans."

"How about next Friday at noon?"

"Didn't you just book the next MAC meeting for that time slot?"

"Oh, yeah, that's right. Okay, make it this coming Monday at 12:30."

"Super." She tagged out and the ER nurse took her place.

"When do you want to do that elective electrical cardioversion?"

"What cardioversion?"

"Mr. Brugada."

"Didn't he decide he didn't want Ontario Hydrotherapy?"

"He telephoned just now to say he's changed his mind."

"Hang on. I'll check."

I called the OR and worked out a date with our anaesthetist. The nurse took down the information and departed. Before I could get out of the Medical Records department our transcriptionist asked me to help her figure out a muffled word on one of her tapes. The mystery word turned out to be "dysphoria." Hmm . . . .

On my way to the medical ward I stole a look at my watch. It was already 9:30 and I hadn't even started rounds yet. Now I had six patients to see, two of whom were allegedly falling apart. Cripes! So much for my carefully laid plans. I was within arm's reach of the door to the ward when the respiratory therapist tackled me.

"Would you be able to help me get approval for a sleep study for Mr. Ondine?"

I don't even recall the details of the conversation. I just remember a sudden moment of clarity in which a single thought crystallized in my mind: *Now I know how those carnival ducks felt.*

When I was a kid, every summer a couple of travelling carnivals would come to our town for a few days. Armed with the contents of our piggy banks, my friends and I would wander through the amazing chaos together. We'd go on all the rides, eat loads of candy and try our luck at the games. One of our favourite games was Shoot the Duck. For a dime you'd get to shoot pellets at a metal duck at the far end of the booth. It was "swimming" from one side to the other, but if you nailed it just right it would spin around and go back in the opposite direction. Each time you hit it a loud *Ding!* would reverberate throughout the booth. *Ding! Ding! Ding! Ding!* It kept trying to get to the other side, but somehow it never made it. Some days I feel like that duck.

Eventually I arrived at the ward. I had just cracked open my first chart when one of the ambulance attendants bellied up to the counter beside me. He looked annoyed.

"So your guy's not DNR anymore," he said.

"That's right."

"You know that means we'll be doing a complete resuscitation on him if he goes sour while we're on the road, right?"

"Go for it."

"Does his family know his code status has been changed?"

I lost it.

"The whole world knows, okay? Go ahead and run a full code! Do a heart transplant if you have to! Just do the goddamn transfer!"

"Okay, okay, take it easy," he muttered. "Just making sure."

I got home at noon with a newfound understanding of the relief Xenophon must have felt when he and his fellow warriors finally clawed their way to the Black Sea. *Thálatta, thálatta! (The sea, the sea!)* I went straight to bed. Sleep claimed me within seconds. Half a minute later the bedside telephone shrilled. I nearly jumped out of my skin.

"Hi, Sweetie," said my wife. "I'm stuck in a meeting and Ellen just called to say she forgot her lunch at home this morning. Do you think maybe you could run it down to the school for her?"

The Simple Math of Medical Errors

Medicine's a tough gig. For one thing, there are so many diseases out there it's almost impossible to learn them all. Although we physicians spend the majority of our time treating a core group of relatively common disorders, we still encounter the bizarre and unexpected often enough to keep us on our toes.

Next, some diseases are protean. It's not uncommon for two people with the same ailment to have entirely different presentations. The converse is also true – unrelated diseases can sometimes generate remarkably similar signs and symptoms.

Another stumbling block is the fact that some patients are poor historians. A portion bury vital clues beneath mountains of irrelevant trivia. When that happens, we have to dig like archaeologists to excavate the information we need. Others have a frustrating tendency to withhold critical details when relating their histories. And then there are always those who just can't seem to remember exactly what it was they came in to see us for. That never portends well.

On the other side of the coin, there are certainly times when we doctors impede the diagnostic process. Sometimes things like being hungry, tired, stressed or swamped reduce our effectiveness. Sometimes we're lazy. Occasionally we develop tunnel vision and fail to consider other potential diagnoses. And sometimes we just plain screw up. How could we not? We're made of the same flesh and blood as everyone else.

In my office I see about 40 patients a day. By the end of most of these encounters I have to make several management decisions. Is this person sick, or not? Is their illness primarily physical or psychological? Do they need investigations? If so, which ones? In what sequence? Within what time frame? Should their medications be adjusted? Do they need to be started on something new? Would they benefit from a visit to an allied health professional or a specialist? What type? How soon? I have approximately 15 minutes to extract an accurate history, perform a relevant examination and come up with a game plan. Does that sound like a tall order? Well, it isn't. It's just business as usual.

In addition to the continuous flow of patients, dozens of reports cross my desk every day. Blood tests, urinalyses, cultures, stool studies, EKGs, x-rays, ultrasounds, CT and MRI scans, bone scans, bone density studies, mammograms, Pap smears, pathology reports, pulmonary function tests, ambulatory blood pressure readings, cardiac monitor reports . . . . The list is endless. As I review each report I have to try to recall why the test was ordered. If the result is normal it can usually be filed away. Significantly abnormal results are flagged and dealt with promptly. Mildly abnormal results are tricky, because they require an answer to the question: Can this be safely filed, or are further investigations required? Not every abnormal test result needs to be acted upon. Part of the art of medicine is knowing when it's appropriate to ignore a result that falls slightly outside the normal range. "Incidentalomas" abound in clinical medicine, and they don't all require a million-dollar workup.

For as long as history has been recorded, most societies have held their healers in high esteem. This respect has usually been accompanied by a certain degree of tolerance vis-à-vis medical errors. We physicians have always been extremely grateful for this unspoken buffer zone of forgiveness. Doctors are human beings, and all human beings make mistakes. If the guy at Domino's makes a mistake, someone could end up getting anchovies instead of mushrooms on their pizza. If I make a mistake, someone could end up dead. It's a terrifying responsibility.

Over the past 30 years there has been a seismic shift in our collective attitude towards mistakes in North America. All of a sudden errors are no longer permissible. Now if something goes wrong, someone has to be held accountable. Our current zeitgeist fosters the belief that if you look hard enough, eventually you'll find someone to blame. Someone to blame equals someone to sue. Successful lawsuit equals big money.

Given the prevailing cultural mindset, it's no surprise the public's tolerance for medical errors has all but evaporated. Nowadays if a physician makes a mistake, there's a fair chance their patient may be more angry than forgiving. Even sympathetic patients are often tempted to initiate litigation when family, friends or the media inundate them with stories of lucrative malpractice settlements. I've seen sweet little old grandmothers morph into near-psychotic greedheads after having been advised what their injury might be "worth." It's not a pretty sight.

Between patient encounters and the interpretation of test results, I estimate I make at least 50 significant decisions a day. Even if I'm right 98 percent of the time (a near-impossibility in clinical medicine), that still means I make one mistake per day. That's a minimum of five a week, or roughly 250 per year.

All of these mistakes are incubating in an increasingly hostile milieu in which highly-informed patients are demanding perfection. Practicing medicine in North America in the 21st century is like juggling hand grenades – no matter how good you are, eventually one of them is going to go off in your face.

* * *

Humble Pie

Buried within the classifieds of our local biweekly newspaper is a small "Thank You" column. In it community members thank one another for various acts of kindness. I receive a handful of these notes every year. Jan and I have a running gag – whenever the latest paper arrives, if there are no messages in it for me she jokes that the "Dr. Gray Thank-You Supplement" must have fallen out again. Pretty droll, but it always makes me laugh.

On those occasions when she mentions there's a note for me, I like to try to guess who sent it before I read it. Over the years I've learned there is surprisingly little correlation between the acuity of the illnesses I treat patients for and subsequent thank-you notes (or lack thereof). Most times it is not patients I literally snatched from the jaws of death who send a note to the newspaper, it's people I assisted in more mundane ways. I never expect to receive thank-you notes, so it brightens my day whenever one comes along. They serve as a reminder that I really am making a difference out here in the trenches.

Mr. Anderson was an 80-year-old patient of mine. He had an acerbic wit and a flawless memory. Although he tended to be fairly cranky with most other health care providers, he always had a good yarn and a devilish wink for me. Unfortunately his body wasn't quite as resilient as his mind, and over time his internal organs began to fail. Despite our best attempts to quell the escalating mutiny, he eventually succumbed to multi-system failure. His death saddened me.

A few days after Mr. Anderson's funeral I was scanning the paper when I came across a thank-you note submitted by his family. It was a long one. In it they thanked several friends of the family, some hospital and Home Care nurses, a couple of ambulance attendants, their minister, the funeral home and the florist. In short, everyone but me.

I'd like to pull a John Wayne and say that the apparent oversight didn't bother me, but it did. I kept thinking: "All those years I worked so hard at trying to keep him healthy and the *florist* gets thanked? Now there's gratitude for you." I grumbled about it all evening. I was still muttering to myself that night as I fell asleep.

When I got to my office the next morning there was a beautiful gift basket waiting for me on my desk. The card attached to it read: "Thank you for your wonderful care of Dad over the years. From the Anderson family."

I felt like a jerk.

Every Breath You Take

Molly was a slightly anxious 40-year-old woman whom I had seen in my office a few times for minor health issues. One morning she presented to the ER intensely short of breath. Her oxygen saturation was only 70 percent and her chest was full of crackles. It took a high-flow oxygen delivery mask to bring her sats back up into the normal range. A chest x-ray was done to help rule out congestive heart failure and pneumonia. To my surprise, it showed extensive scar tissue consistent with a diagnosis of severe pulmonary fibrosis. I admitted her for further investigation.

Pulmonary fibrosis is usually an insidious process. Over the next few days I searched for a reason for her abrupt decompensation. No cause was found. Despite quitting her five-cigarette-a-day smoking habit, she wasn't able to maintain her sats above 90 percent without supplemental oxygen. Arrangements were made for her to have home oxygen as well as an urgent consultation with the nearest available lung specialist. When everything was in place, I discharged her from hospital.

Over the next several months Molly made a number of trips to the respirologist. A lung biopsy revealed progressive pulmonary fibrosis of unknown origin, so she was started on high-dose corticosteroids.

Although she was a pleasant person, Molly had always been a loner who pretty much kept to herself. She was single and had no living relatives. As her shortness of breath worsened, so too did her anxiety. With nowhere else to turn, my office gradually became her main source of support.

The steroids failed to halt the progression of her disease, so immunosuppressants were initiated. When it became obvious that they, too, weren't helping, she was referred further south to a transplant unit in

Toronto. The team there reviewed her case carefully and concluded she was a good candidate for their program. There was only one catch – she would have to move to Toronto. This was not an unreasonable request. Due to the logistics involved in harvesting and transplanting lungs, patients on the waiting list must be able to get to the surgical centre on short notice. Our town was 800 kilometres away from Toronto.

The idea of moving petrified Molly. She agonized over the decision for a long time, but in the end she opted to go. She had no choice, really – to remain at home in our isolated town would have meant certain death.

Packing up and moving to Toronto when you can hardly breathe is no easy feat. It's even more difficult when you have limited savings and no family. True to the spirit of the North, our town came through for Molly. After a lot of searching, a suitable place for her to stay in Toronto was found. A community member whom she barely even knew volunteered to go live with her and provide general assistance. In addition to that, a local service club held a fundraiser to help offset her mounting expenses. Eventually everything was organized and a departure date was set.

A couple of weeks before she was scheduled to leave, Molly came in for an office appointment. Her shortness of breath had worsened and she was feeling overwhelmed. She asked if I could admit her to our hospital until she left for Toronto. I called the medical ward and let them know she'd be coming in.

A fresh battery of tests failed to turn up any new problems. Even so, I didn't think she was well enough to handle a commercial flight. I spoke to the transplant team and they agreed to a direct hospital-to-hospital transfer by jet in one week.

For the next six days I made a point of dropping in and chatting with her for as long as time permitted. If there was no longer anything medical I could do for her, at least I could listen.

At 5:30 on the evening before the transfer a nurse on the medical floor called me at my office to say Molly wanted to speak to me. Apparently she needed to tell me something important. It had been a long day and I was tired. I had already spent 15 minutes with her during my lunch break and I just didn't feel like doing it again. I asked the nurse to tell her I'd see her first thing in the morning before the jet arrived.

Molly died in her sleep at 6:00 a.m. on the morning of her scheduled transfer.

Sometimes at night I lie in bed and wonder what it was she wanted to tell me.

Thank You

It's hard to figure out where the expression "thank you" fits into the practice of modern medicine. Are people obliged to thank me when I help them? Of course not. Would it be nice? Why, yes, it would. Most people do say thanks when I help lighten their load, but a surprising number do not. When I stay up all night struggling to keep a family's loved one alive, I obviously don't expect any sort of material reward, but I don't think it's unreasonable to expect a thank-you.

Now, I know what you're thinking: *"But Slim, it's not like you're treating these people purely out of the goodness of your heart! You're well-paid by the Ministry of Health to provide these services!"*

Yes, I know that. However, I say thanks when the operator puts my call through. I say thank-you whenever the guy at the service station fills my car's tank with gas. I say thanks every morning when the woman at Tim Hortons hands me my bagel and coffee. Should it not therefore be reasonable for me to expect a simple thank-you for treating someone's hemorrhoid, headache or heart attack?

One Sunday afternoon I was paged to the ER *stat*. I raced into the major treatment room to find a screaming 20-month-old boy with multiple second-degree burns all over his body. An older sibling had accidently knocked a kettle off the stove and doused him with boiling water. Large blisters were welling up everywhere and he was in acute distress. He needed immediate fluid resuscitation and pain relief. Unfortunately, he was an unusually chubby little fellow and there were no accessible veins in sight.

A few weeks earlier I had attended a pediatric trauma course and learned about a relatively new way to access the circulatory system of a child. It was called an intraosseous infusion. The technique involves drilling a large bore needle through the shinbone and into the marrow beneath it. Fluids and medications can then be administered directly into the bone marrow. From there they enter the bloodstream. As soon as I got back from the course I ordered some intraosseous kits for our ER. I figured they might come in handy someday.

Several attempts at starting a regular IV were unsuccessful, so I asked one of the ER nurses to open an intraosseous kit. The device consisted of a sharp, hollow, inch-long needle attached to a round, plastic handle. I explained the procedure to the boy's mother. She gave her consent and went outside to wait until we were finished. The nurse immobilized the child for me. While I injected local anaesthetic into his upper shin, I reviewed the procedure in my mind. In the course I had taken we had practised inserting intraosseous needles into inert chicken bones, but this was the real deal – a shrieking, writhing toddler. I pushed the needle firmly into his tibia. When it was solidly embedded I began to twist it in deeper by rotating my wrist from side to side. I could feel the metal grinding its way through the bone. It was a strikingly unpleasant sensation.

Eventually the needle punched through to the marrow. After confirming proper placement we attached it to an IV bag and began infusing morphine and fluids.

As his condition stabilized we inserted catheters and applied dressings to his wounds. I contacted a burn specialist at a pediatric hospital in southern Ontario and had him flown down for definitive care.

Over the next several days we followed his progress via a number of sources, both direct and indirect. By all accounts he was doing very well and was expected to have a satisfactory recovery. We were especially proud to hear the pediatric burn unit had been impressed with the quality of care he had received at our facility. We patted ourselves on the back for a job well done.

The only thing that bothered me slightly about the case was that the mother hadn't thanked me for looking after her child in the ER.

"But Slim, she had other things on her mind! Her son had just been badly burned!"

Yeah, I know. I was there, remember? Although I realize it sounds petty of me to even mention it, I still think a brief thank-you would have been nice. Oh, well. Life goes on.

Exactly one week later I was out in my front yard raking. My daughters were having fun running around and jumping into the piles of leaves. Suddenly an unfamiliar truck pulled up to the curb in front of our house. A man jumped out and strode purposefully across our lawn directly towards me. My kids stopped playing and eyed the stranger cautiously.

"Are you Dr. Gray?"

"Yes."

"I'm Mr. Farquhar. You looked after my son Peyton last weekend when he got burned."

I thought,"Oh, that's who he is! He's dropped by to say thank-you in person! Wow, isn't that considerate?"

He reached into his jacket pocket and pulled out a wad of forms.

"I need these completed ASAP so we can get our travel expenses paid. Can you do them right now?"

I was dumbfounded.
I was enraged.
I was hurt.

"If you drop those off at my office tomorrow morning, I'll see to it they get filled out," I said quietly.

"Sounds good."

He turned around, marched back to his truck and drove off.

Snap!

Last Friday I was on call. During the day the emergency department was hopping. I zipped home at 7:00 p.m. for a quick bite to eat and a 30-minute power nap. At 8:00 I returned to see the evening crop of outpatients. I worked until 11:00 and then charted in Medical Records until midnight. When the paperwork was completed I dropped by the ER to make sure the coast was clear. A pink Post-It note was stuck to my knapsack. Those are never good. This one's *raison d'être* was to advise me that a patient named Mr. Yorke on unit 4 was short of breath and having a rapid pulse. *Geez, how come no one paged me about this?* I went over to the ward to investigate.

As it turned out, Mr. Yorke was one hot mess and I ended up having to work on him for a couple of hours.

At 6:00 a.m. I was summoned back to the ER to stitch up yet another drunken Jethro. This particular genius had taken a swan dive onto a flotilla of empty beer bottles that had spontaneously assembled on his kitchen floor. By the time I finished with him there was hardly any point in trying to go back to bed, so I raided the fridge on unit 4 and ate a couple of mystery-meat sandwiches at the desk. At 8:00 I started my ward rounds. I figured if I got rounds out of the way early I'd be able to enjoy the rest of the day with my family. Of the eight acute and chronic care patients I visited, Mr. Yorke was still the sickest. Our stockroom was fresh out of bags of IV Miracle, so I had to spend another hour or so getting him squared away. By 10:00 I was finished. Freedom! A sunny Saturday and no more work to do!

When I got home I asked my daughters if they wanted to ride their bikes to the park with me. It was looking like the perfect day to fly our new kites. Their answer was a resounding "Yes!" I went upstairs to get ready. Halfway through my shower the phone rang.

"Hello?"

"Hi Dr. Gray. We need a clarification on your order for Mr. Yorke's potassium pills."

After sorting that out I finished getting ready, rounded up the kids and herded them out the front door.

It's not easy riding 15 blocks with a trio of girls ages five, six and seven. I was right in the middle of negotiating a busy intersection when my cell phone started ringing. I shouldered off my backpack and rummaged through its contents until I found it.

"Hello?"

"Dr. Gray, Mr. Yorke is refusing to take his potassium pills."

Suddenly something *snapped*. A severely unhinged stranger who sounded a whole lot like me started caterwauling: **"I don't care! I'm not on call anymore! I did my call day yesterday! Get whoever's on call today to deal with this crap!"**

My kids goggled at me, their mouths hanging open. Passers-by edged away nervously. Small-town family medicine. What's not to like?

Tough Call

One Friday night an elderly patient of mine presented to our emergency department with atypical chest pain. Her EKG had been chronically abnormal ever since a heart attack a few years prior, so it was difficult for the on-call physician to determine whether or not she was experiencing an acute coronary event. He increased her anti-anginal medications and watched her closely. After a period of observation in the ER she was admitted to the medical ward for further monitoring.

When I saw her during my daily inpatient rounds on Saturday morning she was surrounded by a phalanx of concerned family members. Despite the med adjustments, she was still experiencing intermittent low-grade chest discomfort. Her EKGs hadn't changed and her cardiac enzymes were normal. I wanted advice as to how best to proceed with her, so I put in a call to our closest cardiac referral centre.

As luck would have it, my favourite cardiologist was on call. We have a very amicable working relationship, in part because I usually screen my referrals well. Most of the patients I send him ultimately prove to have significant coronary artery pathology. After I went over the details of the case with him he gave me two options: I could continue to manage the patient in our community and send her to his office in a couple of weeks for further workup, or if I was really worried about her I could transfer her to his coronary care unit via air ambulance immediately. It was a generous offer, particularly since her vital signs were rock-solid.

Deep down I knew I could probably soldier on with her a while longer, but my energy levels were low that morning and the thought of trying to unravel yet another medical mystery on what was supposed to be my day off was decidedly unappealing. I was still in the process of figuring out what to do when several of her relatives rushed to the desk to report she was having more chest pain. That did it. I told the cardiologist I'd make arrangements to have her flown down for admission to the CCU.

A week later she dropped in to see me at my office.

"They didn't think it was my heart," she said. "In fact, they discharged me the next day. The cardiologist wants me to have a stress test in a few weeks." I felt a sharp pang of guilt. Not only had I dumped on a colleague, I'd wasted already sparse health care resources by ordering an unnecessary air ambulance transfer. That week her discharge summary from the CCU arrived in the mail. The dictated note was polite, but reading between the lines I could tell the cardiologist was disappointed I had fast-tracked such a non-urgent case.

Three weeks later she had her stress test and passed it with flying colours. I promised myself I'd never bail out like a nervous rookie again. Nobody likes a sieve.

A month later I came in to do rounds on a Sunday morning and discovered a patient of mine had been admitted during the night with a diagnosis of pulmonary edema. Judging from the chart notes Mr. Trapper's course in the ER had been fairly rocky, but things had settled down nicely since his transfer to the ward.

Mr. Trapper was an elderly bachelor with diabetes. He was a cheerful man who liked to crack jokes. When I went to see him he said he was feeling about 75 percent better. On examination, he still had signs of some fluid on his lungs. His EKG showed non-specific changes, and his cardiac enzymes were normal.

As I wrote out his new diet and medication orders I toyed with the idea of calling to request a transfer to the CCU. Although my patient had improved considerably, flash pulmonary edema can sometimes be associated with critical narrowing of a major coronary artery. In addition to that, diabetics are at higher risk for silent ischemia. *Don't be such a wimp*, I told myself. *Look what happened the last time you jumped the gun and flew someone out prematurely. Do you want them to think you've turned into Chicken Little?* I decided to continue managing him at our facility for the time being.

By his fourth day in hospital Mr. Trapper was back to normal. A referral letter requesting outpatient investigations was faxed to the cardiologist. I wrote a prescription for his new medications and arranged for him to see me in my office the following week.

Before he went home I reminded him to call me or return to the hospital if he experienced any further difficulties. He thanked me, packed his belongings into a battered canvas suitcase, and departed.

Mr. Trapper had a massive heart attack and died alone in his cabin a few days later.

So Sue Me

A few years ago I was getting ready to start a shift in the ER when a Code Blue was broadcast on the overhead PA system. I sprinted over to the medical floor. When I got there, a wide-eyed ward clerk pointed mutely at one of the patient rooms. Inside I found three nurses frantically trying to revive an unconscious nine-year-old boy.

Before I had time to ask what had happened, he stopped breathing. I snatched a pediatric ET tube off the crash cart and intubated him. With ventilation his oxygen sats quickly returned to normal. His pulse and blood pressure held steady, so no chest compressions were required. Within minutes most of my colleagues were at the bedside. Together we formulated a differential diagnosis for the respiratory arrest, initiated a course of therapy and contacted a tertiary care centre. A few hours later he was en route to a pediatric ICU via air ambulance.

To our dismay he went into shock and died a few days later. The news decimated us. A pall hung over our hospital for weeks.

I don't often attend patient funerals, but I felt an overwhelming need to go to his. Not surprisingly, the church was packed. The air was so thick with grief it was hard to breathe. I usually have a firm grip on my emotions, but when the deceased child's classmates joined hands and formed a circle around his coffin, I cried.

A few months later I was doing some charting at a workstation in the ER when a briefcase-toting stranger sidled up to me.

"Are you Dr. Gray?" he inquired.

"Yes, I am. How can I help you?"

He fished a manila envelope out of his bag and handed it to me.

"This is for you."

"What is it?"

"Notification."

"Of what?"

"You're being sued for malpractice." He flashed me a jagged smile, turned spryly on his heel and left the department. Talk about *schadenfreude*.

I opened the envelope. Sure enough, it was a lawyer's letter stating the parents of the deceased child were suing two colleagues and me. Having never been sued before, I was stunned. I contacted my legal representative immediately. After carefully analyzing the case, my attorney came to the conclusion I had been included in the lawsuit solely because my name had been recorded in the boy's chart. The fact that the only reason it was there was because I had voluntarily responded to the Code Blue and helped with the resuscitation didn't seem to matter. Apparently, malpractice lawyers like to cast a wide net in order to improve the odds of ensnaring someone. I was advised there was a fair chance I'd eventually be "cut" from the case. There was only one catch – it would take at least a year.

The first six months were sheer misery. My appetite vanished and I lost weight. I couldn't concentrate properly and I developed gruelling insomnia. I reviewed the case in my mind so many times it must have worn a permanent groove into my brain. I could understand the existence of the lawsuit, but why me? What would my family and friends think? What effect would it have on my career? I cycled endlessly between fear and indignation. Sometimes apathy would set in, leaving me feeling hollow and indifferent. I became moody and irritable. Even my kids noticed the change in my behaviour.

In time, the obsessive rumination settled. I started being able to go longer intervals without thinking about the lawsuit. My appetite and sleep improved, and my interest in hobbies slowly began to return. A new steady state was evolving.

Approximately 18 months after my initial notification I received a letter from my attorney stating I had been dropped from the case. No one on the opposing side bothered to apologize for needlessly putting me through hell for a year and a half. I guess my feelings weren't very high on anyone's priority list.

A month later one of the parents of the deceased child telephoned me at my office.

"Dr. Gray?"
"Yes?"
"Can I transfer my family to your medical practice?"
"What?"
"We'd like to switch doctors. Can we start seeing you?"
"I don't think that would be such a good idea."
"Why not?"
"Because you just tried to sue me! You ruined a year of my life!"
"Oh. Okay."

Oddly enough, they called back two weeks later with the exact same request. My answer didn't change.

Earlier this week I was working in the emergency department when we got word a child who had just undergone surgery was having a malignant hyperthermia crisis. As I ran to the OR to assist our anaesthetist, an unexpected thought popped into my head: *For God's sake, don't go in there! If there's a bad outcome, you'll get sued!* I still went, of course.

How can things have been allowed to deteriorate to the point where a qualified physician with training, skills and experience is tempted to not get involved when help is needed?

3:00 a.m.

Most people rarely witness 3:00 a.m., but I see it all the time. I'm a rural physician, so my schedule is frequently out of synch with the rest of society. Due to the small size of our town, it's not unusual for my car to be the only vehicle on the road when I leave the hospital in the dead of night. Driving home alone across a frozen landscape at 3:00 a.m. can be depressing. The complete absence of traffic fuses with the darkness, the drifting snow and my fatigue to create a crushing sense of isolation. Sometimes I feel like I'm the last living person on the planet.

I park in our garage and lug my gear inside. As always, I am struck by how silent the house is at this hour. I hang up my coat and make my way to the kitchen. The supper I missed earlier is waiting for me in the fridge, but it's far too late for me to have a full meal now. In the end I settle for a bowl of cereal. While I eat, I try to read the newspaper. Tonight the stories seem wispy and insubstantial, as if the events described all occurred in a distant universe. I toss the paper into the recycling bin and retreat to the living room. The curtains are open. An arabesque of silver ice crystals garnishes the edges of the picture window. I sit on the piano bench and watch the moonlit snow swirl across our yard.

Eventually I head upstairs. Partway down the hall I stop to check on our daughters. They look so innocent asleep in their beds with their limbs akimbo and their stuffed animals scattered everywhere. After retrieving the cast-off blankets, pillows and toys, I tuck the girls in and give them each a kiss on the forehead. The youngest stirs and awakens. "I love you, Daddy," she murmurs. She hugs me, rolls over and returns to her dreamworld.

It's good to be home.

Carpool Conundrum

Every Monday evening I sit in the subarctic bleachers of our local arena and watch two of my daughters figure skate. Their lesson runs from 6:00 until 7:00. About 10 minutes before the session ends I slip out of the building and drive halfway across town to pick up my third daughter at Beavers. Beavers also finishes at 7:00, which makes retrieving all three of them on time pretty much impossible.

If Beavers happens to wrap up early I try to swoop in, collar Kristen and race back to the arena before Ellen and Alanna get off the ice. Unfortunately, Beavers has a tendency to run late. Even when it does end on time, most nights Kristen doesn't want to leave right away because she's busy touching up her *craft du jour*. As a result, we usually wind up getting back to the arena several minutes after 7:00. Ellen and Alanna don't like it when I'm late, but they try not to complain about it too much because they understand there's no way I can be in two places at the same time. Jan can't bail me out of this weekly predicament, either – she directs the town's community choir every Monday, and as luck would have it, their practices begin at 7:00 p.m. sharp.

One Monday last October I was waiting impatiently for Kristen to finish off her Beavers' Halloween project.

"Come on Kris, we have to go," I said in that voice parents use when we're trying to urge our children to get moving and they're dawdling along as though they have all the time in the world.

"I just need a couple of minutes, Daddy," she pleaded. I checked my watch: 6:59. *The zamboni will be rolling out any second now. Sigh* . . . .

When Kristen was finally finished, she held up her freshly minted Play-Doh sculpture for my scholarly opinion.

"Hey, that looks great, Kris! Ready to go?"

"Okey-dokey."

I helped her gather her belongings. We were just about to make like Elvis and leave the building when I heard an unfamiliar voice call my name. I turned around. A complete stranger was surging across the room towards us. A tiny waif of a girl with pixie-like features trailed in her wake. She looked to be about five years old.

"Hi, I'm Martha!" the woman trumpeted. "We just moved into the house at the end of your street, and our daughter Frieda joined Beavers tonight. My husband drives transport and he's out of town every other Monday. Our car is going to be in the garage for the next few weeks. Would you be able take Frieda to Beavers every second week until we get it back?"

I wasn't sure what to say. Jan usually used my little two-seater sports car to drop Kristen off at Beavers at 6:00 while I took Ellen and Alanna to the arena in the minivan. If I agreed to pick up Frieda then I'd have to transport all four of the children in the van, which would mean I'd need to leave the house earlier and do a double drop-off. As if life wasn't complicated enough already! On the other hand, if I said no I'd look like a selfish *arschloch*. Even if I explained the complexities of our Monday evening schedule to her she'd probably just think I was manufacturing lame excuses. Frieda looked up at me expectantly.

"Sure, that's okay," I said.

"Are you certain it won't be a bother?"

"No bother at all. Will she need a ride next week?"

"Yes, thanks."

"All right, we'll see you next Monday, then."

It's a bit of a pain, but picking up an extra kid every second week for a month or so isn't going to kill me, right?

A week passed and it was Monday evening again. I had assumed Martha would escort her daughter to our house, but when there was no sign of Frieda at 5:50 I dispatched Kristen to go get her. A few minutes later she returned with the wee bairn in tow. Frieda promptly handed me the plastic grocery bag she was carrying.

"My mommy says for you to give this to the ladies at Beavers."

"What's in it?" I asked.

"A list of things I'm allergic to."

"Oh."

"And my EpiPen."

"Okay." Whatever. I ushered the foursome into the van. When they were all settled in I began backing out of the driveway.

"Excuse me?" came a tiny voice from one of the seats behind me.

"Yes, Frieda?"

"I can't do up my seatbelt." I stopped, twisted around, and buckled her in. "Thank you," she said. Very polite, our Frieda.

As we headed to the arena to drop off the skaters, Ellen initiated a conversation with our new ward.

"Hi, my name's Ellen. I'm eight. How old are you?"

"Almost six."

"I'm in grade three. What grade are you in?"

"I don't know."

"What?"

"I don't know."

"How come you don't know what grade you're in?" Ellen asked, puzzled.

"I don't go to school. My mommy teaches my brother and me at home."

"Why?"

"She's afraid if we go to school we'll get beat up."

"Oh."

After the stop at the arena I took Kristen and Frieda to the Scout hall. Kristen and I exited via the van's front doors and waited outside for Frieda. She didn't get out. I reopened my door and stuck my head in to see what the problem was.

"Excuse me?"

"Yes, Frieda?"

"I can't unbuckle my seatbelt." I leaned over and extricated her. "I can't open my door, either." I did the honours. When we entered the hall I delivered Frieda's lengthy allergy scroll and her EpiPen to troop leaders Bubbles and Rainbow. I thought they took it pretty well, considering the fact that they're volunteers, not the staff of a pediatric ICU. They did have one question for me, though: "Did Frieda's mother sign the consent form we sent home last week?"

"What consent form?"

"The one giving the children permission to sing at the nursing home next Monday. See?" She pulled one out of Kristen's coat pocket. Jan had signed it. "If she forgets to send it in, Frieda won't be able to go."

"I'll let her know when I see her later."

After Beavers and skating ended I chauffeured the girls home. When we got to Frieda's house I unbuckled her seatbelt, opened her door and walked her to the front porch. Several knocks later, her mother appeared.

"When you take Frieda next week, don't forget to bring her permission slip for singing at the nursing home," I reminded her.

"Would you mind taking her next week? My husband's going to be out of town again."

"Okay."

After I drove Frieda home the next week she said, "Thank you," and then quickly added: "My mommy said to ask you if I'd be able to get a ride again next Monday."

"Sure Frieda, we'll see you then." She made the same request the following week. And the week after that. And the week after that, too . . . . Finally, one night I went in and asked Martha, "Didn't you say that she'd only need a ride every *second* week?"

"Oh, yes, I did, but since then my husband's schedule has changed. Now he's away every Monday. I hope that's all right with you."

No it's not all right, it's bloody inconvenient!

"Well, I guess so. When did you say your car would be repaired?"

"Um . . . we decided not to go ahead and get it fixed after all. We've put it away for the winter."

Wonderful.

So Frieda became a permanent part of our Monday evening routine. Kristen would fetch her at 5:45. Ellen would buckle her in and off we'd go. You just never knew what little misadventure Frieda was going to have. Most of the time she didn't have her permission slips. She often forgot to wear her winter boots. On the days she did have her boots, she usually forgot to bring her indoor shoes. Once our automatic garage door surprised her and she screeched like a miniature banshee. I'm guessing she had never seen one before. *Amish much?* Another time her mother gave her $15 to bring to the Beaver troop leaders and she somehow managed to lose it during the 30-second walk from her house to ours. That night Jan and I fretted over whether we should pay it for her. Fortunately, Kristen found the missing money on the road the following morning. On one occasion Beavers was held an hour earlier than usual because the hall was going to be used for some other function between 6:00 and 7:00. I notified Martha of the schedule change weeks in advance. The pickup at 5:00 went smoothly. When I returned to drop Frieda off a few minutes past 6:00, her house was dark and deserted. I asked her where she thought her mother might be.

"Probably at church," was her response. *On a Monday night?*

"Which church do you go to?"

"The one with the cross on it."

I had no choice but to take her to the arena with us. Normally I read medical journals while my girls skate. Not that day!

"Excuse me, can I run over there?"

"Sure, Frieda."

Two minutes later: "Excuse me, can I run over there again?"

"Sure."

"Excuse me, can I hop down those stairs?"

"Go for it, Frieda."

"Excuse me, do you think my mom will be home when skating finishes?"

"I sure hope so."

"Excuse me, I'm getting cold."

"Here, Frieda, you can wear my coat."
"Thank you! My hands are cold, too."
"Would you like to borrow my mitts?"
"Thanks!"
"No problem."
"Um . . . ."
"Yes, Frieda?"
"I have to pee."
Sigh . . . .

A couple of months ago Frieda set the record straight regarding the nefarious Harry Potter.
"Excuse me?"
"Yes, Frieda?"
"You know the Harry Potter movie?"
"Yes?"
"It belongs to SATAN."
"What?"
"It belongs to SATAN."
"Well, we sure liked it."
"Oh. Was it funny?"
"Yes, it was."
"Oh. I never saw it."

Last week Frieda's family pulled up stakes and left our small town in search of greener pastures. On the morning of her departure Frieda came over with a batch of freshly baked cookies and a homemade thank-you card. Inside the card was a crayon drawing of me and four little girls driving down the road in a minivan. The girls were all holding hands, and everyone looked happy. Even the sun was smiling.

We're going to miss you, Frieda.

Chiaroscuro (*Light and Dark*)

What's worse, preparing incessantly for a war that never comes, or maintaining a state of blissful ignorance and getting caught flat-footed when the bombs start falling?

Educating my daughters about racism may help reduce its sting when they finally encounter it firsthand, but it will also hasten their loss of innocence. I've always been of the opinion that if my kids have to learn certain unpalatable truths about race relations, I'd rather they get the facts from me than from some bozo on the playground. I can mete out the required information in carefully measured doses, which is obviously far superior to having someone unexpectedly dump the entire toxic payload on them in one fell swoop.

Gradual desensitization makes more sense than abrupt immersion, doesn't it? Sure it does. Unless . . . . Unless the anticipated immersion never occurs. What if I'm preparing them for something that's never going to happen?

I'm black and my wife is white. Although our three daughters are of mixed racial heritage, history tells us that society will view them as black. Jan and I aren't sure about how best to prepare them to cope with racism. I favour taking a no-holds-barred, worst-case-scenario approach and teaching them everything up front. She prefers the concept of letting them gradually come to their own conclusions.

I don't want my daughters to develop an unnecessarily jaundiced view of the world, but I don't want to see them get blindsided, either. What's better, idealism or pragmatism? Should I hope for the best or plan for the worst? Tough choices. But then, no one ever said parenting was going to be easy.

Lost in Translation

"What we've got here is failure to communicate."
– Captain, Road Prison 36, *Cool Hand Luke*

I have a patient named Irmgard who doesn't speak any English. The first time I saw her in the office she brought her friend Roy to translate. The conversation went something like this:

"Hi, I'm Dr. Gray."

"Roy." He shook my hand, then pointed at his comrade. "Irmgard," he said. She waved. I waved back.

"Could you please ask her what's wrong today?"

They conversed in their language for a while, then Roy turned to me and said something like: "Hibida bibida pain hibida vonch stomach hibida shrek tang two weeks."

"What?"

"Hibida bibida pain hibida vonch stomach hibida shrek tang two weeks."

"Um . . . She's been having pain in her stomach for two weeks?"

"Yes."

"Has she ever had this before?"

They spoke again. He looked at me and shook his head, "No."

"Has she had any change in her weight or blood in her stools?"

They conferred. At length he told me: "Hibida bibida same stretch munch nona lollapalooza."

"What?"

It was starting to look like I'd soon be needing a translator for my translator.

"Did anyone in her family ever have bowel cancer?"

They had an animated discussion that went on for a full minute. I fidgeted in my seat and waited. *Patience, Grasshopper*. Finally Roy swivelled around to face me and relayed her answer: "Purple."

I made a mental note to never use Roy as a translator again.

Patients Say The Darndest Things!

"Yesterday I went to the hospital and they did a PAP test on my throat."

"What's your pain like?"
"It's magnetic."

"Does it hurt anywhere?"
"In bits and pieces."

"How high are your blood sugars?"
"Anywhere from 4-foot-7 to 6-foot-5."

"What's your diarrhea like?"
"It's kind of juicy."

"How bad is your pain on a scale of one to 10?"
"Not too bad – about a nine."

"Hey, doc, would you be able to fill out this welfare form for me?"
"Okay. What's your medical reason for not being able to work?"
"Umm . . . I don't really have one."

"My vision's blurry, doc."
"Did you see an optometrist?"
"Yes."
"What did they say?"
"She gave me some new glasses."
"Do they help at all?"
"They work great, but I keep forgetting to wear them."

"I was watching television the other day and they said those cholesterol pills you put me on do something to the lining of the wall."
"The wall of what?"
"I dunno; I wasn't paying that much attention."

"What's your last name?"
"Vogl."
"Is that European?"
"No, it's German."

"Don't inject me with that cortisone stuff, doc. Twenty years ago they injected some in my wrist and it stiffened up so bad I could hardly use it!"
"That's odd. Why did they do the injection in the first place?"
"It was getting stiff."

"Did anyone in your family develop heart disease at a young age?"
"Yes, my great-grandmother."
"How old was she when she started having heart trouble?"
"97."

Certified drug seeker:
"Geez, doc, I'm taking *way* too many Tylenol 3s. Can I get some morphine instead?"

Teenager who's been slouching around the waiting room playing Game Boy, eating Cheezies and listening to his iPod:
"I have a stomach ache."
"How bad is your pain on a scale of one to 10?"
"17."
"The maximum possible score is 10."
"Oh, okay, I get it. Um, let's see . . . I guess it's about a 12, then."
"The number can't be any greater than 10, and a 10 would be like someone cutting your leg off with a rusty chainsaw."
"Oh. Well in that case it's a 9½."

. . . and sometimes sleep-deprived nurses say the darndest things!
"Mr. Bryant, since you're having trouble peeing I'm going to put this catheter in you, okay?"
"Does it go in my nose?"
"Do you pee through your nose?"

Let's Get Physicals

"I'm here for my yearly complete examination."
"I think the wife booked me for a checkup."
"I'm fine, but I need a physical for my class A-Z driver's license."
"I want to be tested for *everything*."
"Can you book me for one of those total body scan things?"

The complete physical begins with a series of health-related questions called the review of systems. The goal of these questions is to ferret out occult disease. In my experience, patients' responses tend to be influenced by two main things – their personality type and the reason for the physical.

On the one hand are healthy people who are seeing me solely because they need to have their mandatory job-related physical examination forms filled out. On the rare occasion that they actually do have an active medical problem, they go to great lengths to hide it from me. It's not too difficult to figure out why – their livelihood depends on my giving them a clean bill of health. In these patients, the system reviews are shockingly brief:

"Have you been having any chest pain?"

"No."

"Shortness of breath?"

"No."

"Weight loss?"

"No."

"Wait a minute – according to our scale, you've lost 40 pounds over the past three months."

"Really? I hadn't noticed. Probably just that stomach flu I had last week. Hey, how about those Winnipeg Jets!"

Neurotics who are in for "a good physical" represent the other side of the equation:

"Have you been having any chest pain?"

Mr. Somatoform gets that far-away look in his eyes. He strokes his chin thoughtfully as he contemplates the question.

"Now that you mention it, I did have an episode of chest pain not that long ago."

"When?"

"Last Christmas."

"Nine months ago?"

"Yes."

"What sort of pain was it?"

"It felt like a bolt of lightning."

"Where did you feel it?"

"It shot from my right armpit to the centre of my chin."

"How long did it last?"

"About three-quarters of a second."

"Has it ever come back?"

"No, it hasn't. What do you think it was, doc? Could it have been a heart attack? Should I be seeing a cardiologist?"

"I don't know what it was, but I'm pretty sure it wasn't anything too serious. Let's move on. Have you had any shortness of breath?"

"Funny you should mention that . . . ."

Ramblers are a breed unto themselves:

"Have you been having any chest pain?"

"Chest pain, chest pain . . . . I'm not quite sure how to answer that, doctor. I haven't had any chest pain *lately*, but back in the winter of '64 old doc Tilley had to admit me to the hospital for two days on account of the fact I was getting a mighty peculiar discomfort – I can't really say it was a pain, mind you, because it was more of an ache than an actual pain, sort of like a nagging toothache, if you know what I mean – right above this here rib. At first they thought it might be pleurisy because plenty of folks in our neck of the woods had been coming down with it right around the same time I took sick, but in the end doc Tilley figured it was just . . . uh . . . doctor?"

"Zzzzzzz . . . ."

And let's not forget the Chronically Vague:

"Have you been having any chest pain?"

"Uh-huh."

"How long have you been getting it?"

"Huh?"

"How long have you been getting the chest pain?"

Mr. Isidore gazes at me with the eyes of a chicken. After half a minute of deep thought he responds, "Quite a while."

"How long is 'quite a while'?"

"Oh, I dunno. A long time."

"Weeks? Months? Years, perhaps?"

"I dunno. Been quite a while, though."

After I've completed the review of systems I usually leave the room while the patient changes into a gown. If I return to find they've put the gown on with the gap facing the front instead of the back, I automatically deduct two points. The same applies to people who still have their T-shirt on underneath the gown.

I start every physical by asking my patient to turn their wrist over so I can palpate their radial pulse. Due to the location of the artery, it's easier for me to check the right wrist than the left. Inexplicably, 98 percent of patients offer me their left wrist. Why is that? I'm sure there's a research paper for some starving university student in there somewhere. Similarly, when I examine patients' necks I usually ask them to tilt their heads downward slightly to make it easier for me to feel the glands. Most people immediately hyperextend their neck, which results in them staring up at the ceiling. Go figure.

Some people have more earwax than Shrek. Every so often I come across an unexpected surprise, like the time I discovered a bunch of uncooked spaghetti noodles wedged into a young man's ear canal. As it turned out, earlier that week he had used them in an unsuccessful attempt to curette out some earwax. Epic fail! Once I had to flush a fly out of someone's ear canal. How the frak do you get a fly in your ear?

When the ear exam is finished, I'm ready to inspect the throat. I stand in front of my patient, aim a flashlight at their mouth and ask them to open wide. Three-quarters of people open their eyes widely instead of their mouth. Research paper!

Occasionally a detailed eye exam is required. Some people are unbelievably calm when it comes to having their eyes checked – irritating drops and dazzling lights shone directly into their pupils don't faze them in the slightest. Others are eye wimps – the instant the ophthalmology tray is brought out they reflexively scrunch their eyelids shut so tightly a crowbar couldn't pry them open. It usually takes a fair bit of cajoling before these folks will allow me to proceed. Years of examining eyes have taught me that there are four cardinal directions: up, down, left and the other left. "Okay, Mrs. Carter, please look to your left. No, the other left."

Next comes the throat. When I push down on someone's tongue with ye olde glorified Popsicle stick and ask them to say "ah," it's not because that's how I get my jollies. Saying "ah" makes the soft palate rise, which makes it easier for me to visualize the back of the throat. Half the time I ask patients to say "ah," they either straight-up don't do it or else they try to fake it. What? Do they think I won't notice? Hel-*lo*, McFly, I'm right here! I notice! Say "ah!"

I just love it when someone a foot and a half away from me spontaneously ejects their dentures to show me a lesion in their mouth. Isn't there some sort of unwritten rule of social conduct that stipulates prior to popping out one's false teeth, a person is supposed to give innocent bystanders fair warning? I'm still waiting for the day somebody asks me to hold their drippy dentures for them.

Chest auscultation is always interesting. When asked to take deep breaths, many people take one deep breath and hold it. How is that supposed to help me? Sometimes I'm tempted to sit back and wait to see how long they'd last. And then there are the times when patients seem to forget how to breathe and I end up having to remind them to exhale after each inspiration. "Deep breath . . . exhale! Deep breath . . . exhale!" When I get tired of repeating myself I say, "That's good! Just keep doing that, okay?" Seems to work.

While I'm on the topic, what mysterious force compels people to start talking to me while I'm auscultating their chest with my stethoscope? At least once a day I'll be straining to decipher a subtle heart sound when suddenly "**My great-grandmother died of a heart attack when she was 98!**" explodes into my eardrums. Now *that's* annoying. Minus 10 points.

The umbilicus is the centre of the abdomen. Heck, it's practically the centre of the entire body. You'd think people would make an attempt to keep it clean, right? Maybe even treat it to a little soap and water once in a while? Don't count on it. I'm here to tell you that the hygienically-challenged walk among us. Some belly buttons are so full of dirt, you could plant an oak tree in them. Others contain enough lint to fill a Beanie Baby. Wash your belly buttons, people! *This has been a public service announcement . . . .*

Centuries ago, when I needed to evaluate male patients for groin hernias I would insert my gloved finger into their inguinal canal and ask them to cough. This inevitably resulted in them coughing all over me. Nowadays I say, "Please cover your mouth and cough." My patients often look a little baffled when I make this request. Maybe they're thinking, "You mean I don't get to cough on you anymore? Bummer!"

Sooner or later all good things must come to an end. Once the examination is over we discuss my findings as well as any recommended investigations and treatments. When we're finished most people say thanks, walk out and shut the door behind them. I'm never quite sure why they close the door. Perhaps they think I plan to teleport out of the room. Fortunately, I'm not claustrophobic. I finish my charting, reopen the door and mosey on down the hall to see what new challenges await me.

Survey Says . . . .

My desk is littered with surveys. We rural physicians are a hot research topic these days – everyone wants to know what makes us tick. I imagine the brainiacs in their think tanks across the nation scratching their heads, vexed and perplexed.

"What makes them venture beyond city limits?" they ask one another. "And more importantly, what keeps them out there?" More fruitless head-scratching. Suddenly one of them leaps to his feet. He looks excited. Head Boffin arches a bushy eyebrow in the direction of his impulsive young colleague.

"Yes?"

"Sir, I've got it! Let's send them all surveys!"

"Surveys?"

"Yes! We'll ask them each a few hundred questions and then have our quantum computers analyze their responses!"

Head Boffin nods; slowly at first, then with increasing enthusiasm. Finally he breaks into a wide grin.

"Splendid idea, Dilton! First class! We'll start immediately."

And so it begins.

My receptionist unceremoniously dumps the morning mail onto my already overflowing desk. Junk, bills, test results, insurance forms, more bills . . . and two objects that look suspiciously like surveys. Shoulders sagging, I open the first one.

"Dear doctor, we truly appreciate you dedicating your life to rural medicine *yada yada yada* and we hope you won't mind filling out the enclosed survey. Please review the following 200 items and rate their importance in terms of the impact they have on your desire to continue practicing rurally. We estimate this survey should take you no longer than 45 minutes to complete." *What?!* 45 minutes? Are they nuts? I'll be lucky if I get 10 minutes for lunch today! I wad the oversized monstrosity into a ball and three-point it into the recycling bin across the room. *The crowd goes wild* . . . .

Item two is a follow-up letter from a group whose survey I completed a few weeks ago. As I recall, this particular survey had asked more personal questions than most, but its authors had gone to great lengths to assure that all responses would be held in the strictest confidence. They also promised names would not be linked to the forms, so it would be impossible for them to trace answers back to the individual respondents.

"Dear Dr. 655, thank you very much for taking the time to fill out our survey. We notice, however, that you neglected to answer questions 19 and 99. Please complete them and return the form to us in the enclosed self-addressed envelope."

Okay, this I can handle. I quickly finish off the questionnaire and drop it in the outgoing mail tray. Several hours later the penny drops – if they claim to be incapable of tracking the doctors filling out their surveys, how did they know the incomplete one was mine? Egads! I've been duped! With my luck the study will turn out to be the product of some nebulous federal intelligence-gathering agency. Good thing I didn't mention my fluffy pink slipper fetish in the "deviant tendencies" section . . . or did I?

Although surveys can be a real nuisance, I'll probably continue to fill out the shorter ones for years to come. Why? I figure those poor research eggheads need all the help they can get in their noble quest to decode the enigma of the rural physician. If they eventually succeed, perhaps one day we'll be featured on a segment of *Hinterland's Who's Who*. First will come the familiar, haunting flute melody, followed by that unnaturally calm voiceover: *"The Canadian rural physician is a peculiar beast that appears to thrive on challenge and adversity. Only recently have scientists come to understand why this curious creature voluntarily makes its home in the underpopulated nether regions of our great land . . . ."*

Prescription for Parenting Skills

A few months ago one of my patients brought her three-year-old son in to see me. Although little Genghis had only recently begun attending daycare, the workers there were so alarmed by his pervasive aggression and impulsiveness they insisted he be assessed by a physician ASAP.

I walked in to find the rambunctious little fellow gleefully dismantling my examination room. His mother seemed oblivious to the crime scene unfolding around her. After reining him in a bit I obtained a history and wrestled my way through a physical. By the time I was finished, ADHD and suboptimal parenting were highest on my list of potential diagnoses. I spent several minutes reviewing my findings with his mother, gave her some reading material and made arrangements for a follow-up visit.

As I was about to leave I remembered Genghis had a five-year-old brother who had always struck me as being excessively busy. The last time I saw him I had suggested we schedule an appointment to explore the matter further, but his parents hadn't taken me up on the offer.

"Did Anakin start school this year?"

"Yes, he did."

"How's he making out?"

"Super!"

"I'm glad to hear that." I began leaking towards the door.

"At first we were getting a lot of notes from his teachers about his behaviour, but a few weeks ago I figured out a way to stop that."

"How?"

"I just give him some Gravol right before he leaves for school every morning. It works great – he hasn't brought home a single note since!"

Introspect/*Apologia*

Lately I've been reviewing my medical narratives. Some are autobiographical, others reflect patient encounters, and most of the remainder relate to parenting. One thing I've noticed is that a few of the vignettes depicting my interactions with patients are slightly cynical. Usually it's just my warped sense of humour at play, but once in a while there's a bit of an edge to it. Some of this can probably be attributed to representational bias. I'm no neurobiologist, but I suspect difficult experiences engender higher rates of memory protein synthesis than neutral events. In addition to that, stories involving conflict are intrinsically more interesting to write about and analyze than their more peaceful counterparts. Who wants to read a book about unicorns frolicking in the sunset? For the purposes of discussion, though, if we suppose that I do in fact have an embryonic case of misanthropy gestating, is it being nourished by my patients, my job, or me? I think it's probably a combination of all three.

For starters, I am definitely not the touchy-feely type. I tend to favour a linear, problem-solving approach to medicine. Within the first few minutes of most interviews I've usually assigned my patient's presenting complaint to one of four categories:

1) I can fix this.
2) I can't fix this myself, but I know someone who can.
3) I'm not exactly sure what's going on here, but I get the impression it's something fixable.
4) Jesus and Gandalf combined couldn't fix this.

The instant I realize I'm probably not going to be able to help the person I'm seeing in any meaningful way, I start getting fidgety. The way I see it, every morning I arrive at work with a finite amount of expendable energy. Once it's used up, I'm pretty much done for the day, psychologically speaking. This means I have to ration my resources wisely in order to try to do the greatest good for the greatest number of people. There's nothing esoteric about this – it's basic Utilitarianism 101. Unfortunately, a small percentage of patients are like black holes – they'll pull you over their event horizon and suck all the energy out of you in a single sitting if you allow it. Trying to help them is akin to watering the Sahara with a garden hose. Over the years I've treated a number of these unusually needy people. It's been my experience that no matter what I do for them, no matter how much time I spend, they never seem to get significantly better. Working with this challenging subgroup requires a lot of patience. Unfortunately, patience is not one of my strong suits. In fact, some days it seems I have none at all. This regrettable character flaw of mine undoubtedly contributes to the frustration felt on both sides of the desk from time to time.

I also have some difficulty dealing with the fraction of patients I classify as canaries. What's the story behind the term? Coal miners of yesteryear often brought caged canaries underground with them for use as low-tech early warning systems. Canaries were known to be disproportionately sensitive to methane and carbon monoxide. This made the birds ideal harbingers - if a canary suddenly stopped chirping and belly-flopped off its perch, the miners knew it was time to get the hell out of Dodge. Poor canaries. Always the first to keel over whenever the environment is anything less than perfect.

Another obstacle stems from the fact that although I'm always hoping to receive a reasonably concise, coherent history, sometimes all I'm offered is a vague mishmash that meanders all over the place. At the end of some of the more tangential interviews I leave the room wondering if I just went through the looking-glass again. I need to work on not getting so bent out of shape when the story being related to me is more circuitous than I'd prefer.

According to the *True Colors* personality test, I'm off the scale at the gold-green end of the spectrum. This means I'm analytical and organized to the max. The good news is that these are both useful traits when it comes to things like running an efficient office practice or maintaining control of an ER that's trying to go nuclear. Unfortunately, my high scores in these areas come largely at the expense of the orange-blue characteristics, namely impulsivity and empathy. I can manage just fine without the impulsivity, but a little more compassion would certainly be a plus, especially considering my chosen profession.

What else am I guilty of? Misdemeanours, mostly. I'd probably quit my job tomorrow if I won the 6/49 jackpot, so I'm guessing that means I'm no Mother Teresa. I'm chronically late. I biorhythm down to zero at about 10:00 every morning. I get crotchety when I'm tired. I'm set in my ways. I'm a tad OCD. I get antsy when I can't logic things together. I have a tendency to display exit-seeking behaviour during futile patient interviews, particularly those of the asymptotic variety. And sometimes I can't help but wonder if my helping keep certain individuals healthy and reproducing is a direct violation of Darwin's law of natural selection.

Lastly, there's the matter of my smouldering cynicism. For the past couple of years it's been quietly modifying my worldview. I don't think cynicism is chic. I agree with Bruce Mau, founder of the Massive Change Network, when he says that anyone can be cynical, but it takes guts to be optimistic. Nevertheless, I suspect I'm losing the battle. I think part of the reason I'm getting jaded stems from the fact that every day I observe people taking advantage of the system. To make matters worse, not only do I have to witness it, I'm often conscripted into helping them do it. How does this happen, you may wonder? Due to the nature of my job, I have the power to grant certain things. I never asked for this privilege – it comes with the title and there's no way to divest myself of it. Modern-day family physicians have somehow been transformed into living cornucopias expected to generate an infinite supply of sympathetic off-work slips, welfare letters, disability pensions, tax credit papers, insurance forms, subsidized housing recommendations, accessible parking permits, travel grants, etc. This, of course, is in addition to the usual prescriptions, tests, referrals, and so on. After a while the endless stream of requests starts to wear you down. Usually the things I'm asked to provide are fair and reasonable. Sometimes . . . not so much. I try to be as accommodating as possible, but I do have to draw the line somewhere. Whenever I say no, conflict ensues. Here are some of the less reasonable requests I've had to deal with over the past few months:

1. A patient asked me to provide her with a prescription for foot orthotics. She had been seeing an alternative health care professional for sore feet for several months and in the end he fashioned her a $400 pair of shoe inserts. Her insurance company refused to reimburse the money unless the inserts had been ordered by an MD, so she dropped in to inform me I needed to write a prescription for them. The catch is she had never seen me for that particular problem before. She ended her request with ". . . and make sure it's dated before June 5th, because that's when I submitted the claim." What should I do? If I agree, I'm participating in a low-grade swindle. If I refuse, I'm labelled mean-spirited and difficult. I guess you could

say the money's not coming out of my pocket, so why should I care, but it just doesn't seem right.

2. Someone with mild quasi-depressive symptoms who has repeatedly eschewed offers of counselling asked for a note stating it was medically necessary for him to take a paid six-month leave of absence so he could "rest up a bit."

3. A fellow who bumped his head at work two years ago and hadn't mentioned any problems related to the accident since it occurred came in to see me. He had recently been laid off, so he'd decided to launch a Worker's Compensation claim over the incident. He wanted an MRI of his head, neck, shoulders and back as well as a referral to a neurologist "right away."

4. A few people with no particular musculoskeletal disorders asked that letters be sent to their insurance companies informing them that in my opinion it was medically necessary for them to have prolonged courses of massage therapy at their chiropractor's office. "It's covered under our plan, so we might as well get our money's worth."

5. A fit senior who hikes and rides his mountain bike all over the place insisted I sign a form stating he is too disabled to walk in order to allow him to qualify for an income tax disability credit. He was surprisingly irate when I declined.

6. A patient wanted me to send a letter to the town's subsidized-rental housing administrator saying I felt it was imperative she and her equally able-bodied spouse be given the next available ground floor apartment. Why? "We don't like stairs."

7. A squadron of shady transients drifted into town looking to score prescriptions for OxyContin, fentanyl patches, sedatives and other goodies. Don't even get me started on those con-artists – in the Periodic Table of Society, ER drug seekers are plutonium!

8. One of my patients showed up at the office saying he'd missed

the preceding week of work due to a bad cold. He assured me he was fine now, but he needed a return to work note to present to his employer in order to collect his sick pay. Neither I nor any of my colleagues had seen him during the week he was off, so there was no objective way to corroborate his story. This isn't the first time he's pulled this stunt. How do I know he wasn't out moose hunting with his buddies?

9. Another patient had some money locked into a GIC. In order to withdraw the funds prematurely without incurring the standard financial penalties he wanted me to advise his bank that it was medically necessary for him to get his money right away. The reason he needed the money in such a hurry? He wanted to buy a new snowmobile.

10. And the grand prize winner:
"Can I get a letter saying you feel it's necessary for my health for me to have carpets installed in my apartment?"
"Why?"
"I like carpet!"

I wonder what a prescription for carpet would look like?

Pssst . . . Want to Buy Some Medical Products?

A couple of months ago I was in the middle of doing a Pap test when my receptionist knocked on the door.
"Donovan? There's a Dr. Julep from Ottawa on the line for you."
"Who?"
"Dr. Julep from Ottawa. She says it's very important."
"Okay, I'll be right there." I handed my nurse the cervical brush and hurried out of the room. "Hello?"
"Hi Dr. Gray. Listen, I really liked that story you wrote for the *Medical Post* about drug seekers in the ER."
"Uh, thank you. What did you say your name was again?"

"Dr. Mint Julep."

"Do I know you?"

"No, I don't believe we've ever met. Dr. Gray, in light of the recent tragedy in Walkerton, do you have any concerns about the condition of the drinking water in your town?"

"What?"

"As a respected health care professional in your community, you could be generating a substantial amount of additional income by selling high-quality home water purification systems."

"What?"

"You could offer them to the patients in your practice. I guarantee you, they'd sell like hotcakes."

"Are you serious?"

"We also have an exceptional line of vitamins, tonics and natural products."

"Let me get this straight – you want me to use my office to peddle the medical equivalent of Amway?"

"Our products are of the highest calibre and –"

"Goodbye!" *Click!*

Last week I got a phone call from Montreal. This time I was prepared.

"Good afternoon, Dr. Gray! This is Dr. McQuack. Loved your article on cancer in the *Medical Post*."

"Do I know you?"

"Ah, no, but Dr. Gray, is it safe for me to assume you have a genuine interest in the health and well-being of cancer patients?"

"No."

"Uh . . . but that article you wrote . . . ."

"I made it all up."

"Really?"

"Yep."

"Um, well, anyway we offer several lines of very exclusive biloba vera colonics as well as specially enhanced carrot juice enemas that have been scientifically proven to put most cancers into permanent remission – "

"As a matter of fact, I don't even like cancer patients."

"But – "
"Have a nice day!" *Click!*

Sahara Mouth

I once had a sweet little old lady in my practice who complained bitterly of having dry eyes. None of the regular treatments for dry eyes seemed to have the slightest effect on her. I began to wonder if she might have Sjögren's syndrome, a condition in which autoimmune destruction of the salivary and lacrimal glands leads to chronic dryness of the mouth and eyes. It's possible to have either problem in isolation, but usually the two coexist. Every month or two when she came to see me at my office I'd ask, "Do you have a dry mouth?"

"No."

"Are you sure?"

"Positive. No dry mouth, doctor."

After a couple of years of unsuccessfully battling this mysterious affliction I finally said uncle and sent her to a newly-launched dry-eye specialty clinic at a teaching hospital in Toronto. A few weeks later the consultant's letter arrived. The opening lines read: "This pleasant 80-year-old woman presents complaining of a two-year history of dry eyes and dry mouth. She says she has to suck on hard candy almost continuously in order to relieve the mouth dryness." *What the hell?* The consultant went on to conclude: ". . . a fairly obvious case of Sjögren's syndrome." I was gobsmacked. I requested my patient be called in for an appointment *pronto*.

When she arrived she was grinning from ear to ear. She happily displayed the bottle of Salagen the specialist had prescribed for her.

"This works great! Those doctors in Toronto, they sure know what they're doing," she remarked ever so thoughtfully.

I got straight to the point.

"Mrs. Kareishu, how come you always told me your mouth wasn't dry?"

"Well, my mouth feels moist when I suck on a hard candy, so

since I'm just about always sucking on one, it never really gets dry!"

My eyes rolled up with such force I was nearly knocked out.

Beginner's Luck

Recently Jan and I accompanied a group of friends from our town to a Supertramp concert in a nearby city. When the show ended, someone suggested we check out the local casino. I had never been to a casino before. My mind conjured up Hollywood-inspired images of beautiful people, laughter and glittering roulette wheels. Hey, that sounded like fun! We hopped into our vehicles and headed out to The Slots.

The lot was jam-packed, so it took us a while to find parking spots. When we finally got into the lobby the first thing I noticed was a sign stating any patrons found leaving their children unattended in the parking lot would be banned from the premises for five years. There were also several posters for Gamblers Anonymous and Ontario Addiction Services on the walls. Hmm . . . .

We decided to go watch the horse races. There were a few hundred spectators at the downs. A huge scoreboard above the racetrack updated the odds continuously. One of our friends had a little gambling experience, so he gave us a crash course on how to bet on horses. Perhaps I misunderstood him, but it sounded to me like I could either bet on the favourite and win a pittance, or bet on one of the long shots and lose my shirt. It seemed like an expensive way to have a good time.

After watching pint-sized jockeys whip their tired steeds around the track for half an hour we lost interest and returned to the main building. By then I was getting pretty hungry, so I asked one of the employees where the restaurant was. He advised me the cafeteria was the only place where food could be purchased. I went in and looked around. They had every species of Cheezies, Pringles and Doritos known to man, but no hot meals or sandwiches. Oh, well. It was time to get the show on the road. We hurried down the main hallway, past a knot of beefy security guards and into the casino.

It was like stepping into *The Twilight Zone*. Hundreds of slot machines filled the room, and nearly all of them were occupied. The glassy-eyed zombies playing the slots were pushing buttons and pulling levers like well-trained lab rats. Whenever the credit on their machines ran out, most people automatically pulled out a fresh bill and carried on playing. Some of them were using $100 bills. Every other player had a cigarette in hand. Once in a while they'd stop pushing buttons long enough to take a drag. The air was blue with smoke.

I took a stroll around the room. Most people looked as though they didn't have a lot of disposable income. There were markedly few conversations taking place, and no one was laughing. Everyone seemed to be grimly fixated on their slot machine. I noticed several players wearing necklaces with a credit card-type device attached to them. The cards were inserted into a special groove located on the front of each machine. I asked a waitress what they were for.

"Oh, those are frequent player cards. It works kind of like Air Miles. The card keeps track of how much you play. The more you play, the more points you get. When you accumulate enough points you can trade them in for things like food or free lottery tickets. Would you like me to get you one?"

"No, thank you," I replied. I backed away from her warily.

There were no seats for non-players in the room. Your options were to play, stand around and get lung cancer, or leave. I decided to play.

I found a vacant one-armed bandit, sat down and fed it $20. My cash was instantly converted into 80 credits. It reminded me of something I once read in a psychology textbook: Converting money into more abstract things like poker chips or "credits" tends to make people less inhibited about spending it. Someone showed me how to work the device. Essentially, all I had to do was press one button to indicate the quantity of money I wanted to bet, then either press a second button or pull down the lever to make the icons spin. If a winning combination lined up I'd be awarded credits; otherwise credits would be deducted. I could cash out at any time. It seemed straightforward enough. I started pressing buttons.

Press, press, look.

Press, press, look.

Not exactly the most intellectual game going, but frighteningly enough there was an undeniable appeal to it. It was sort of like participating in a lottery – even though you were fully aware the odds of winning big were almost zero, each time you pressed that second button you felt like this *could* be the time you won the jackpot.

I must have been having a bit of beginner's luck, because 15 minutes later I was up to 120 credits. The Vulcan in me spoke up: *Now would be a logical time for you to quit and cash out a winner.*

"Are you kidding? I'm on a roll! Nothing can stop me now!"

But the odds are stacked against you, so if you play long enough, you'll be guaranteed to lose.

"No way, killjoy - I'm red hot! I'm going all the way!"

Suit yourself.

I continued playing.

Five minutes later I was down to 30 credits. A waitress came by.

"Would you like a drink, sir?"

I hesitated. Drinking and gambling are two activities that probably should not be combined.

"No, thank you."

"Coffee and pop are free," she added.

"Do you have decaf?"

"No."

I knew if I had a cup of regular coffee this late at night I'd be up for hours. I'm sure there's nothing a casino likes better than an insomniac playing one of their slot machines.

"No thanks." As she turned to go I asked, "Any idea what time it is?"

"Sorry, I don't have a watch."

I caught a glimpse of the wrist of another casino employee who happened to be passing by. No watch. I scanned the walls. There wasn't a single clock in the entire room. There were no windows, either – all the lighting came from artificial sources. Background music was curiously absent. The only sound was the trance-like drone of the slot machines. It was almost hypnotic. No clocks, no windows, perpetual light and continuous white noise. Whoever designed this room obviously wanted to make its occupants as oblivious to the passage of time as possible. The Room That Time Forgot. Talk about the ultimate gambling environment. I returned to my game.

A short while later my credits ran out. Without even thinking, I fished out another bill. I was about to slide it in when my inner Vulcan murmured: *Are you sure you want to go down this road?*

I thought about it for a spell, then stood up.

The player to my right squinted at me dully. I noted with some disquiet that we bore a passing resemblance. In addition to looking like he was half in the bag, he was tethered to his machine by one of those creepy Frequent Gambler umbilical cords. I wondered if somewhere out there a family was waiting for him to come home. Hoping and waiting. Night after night.

"Ya done already?" he slurred.

"Yep."

"Well, dat's how it goes, eh? Ya put yer money in da @$#% machine, ya press da button and it eats yer @$#% money!" He leaned over to my freshly vacated slot machine, dropped a couple of tokens in and pulled down the lever. Three different icons tumbled into place. He shrugged, turned back to his own unit and resumed playing.

Out-bluffing the Kids

Our friend Gord is an ER doc in a nearby city. Last winter we invited him to visit us in our small town. One of the things he and his two sons mentioned they wanted to do during their stay with us was go sledding. A few hours before they arrived, Jan inspected our sliding paraphernalia. The crazy carpets were fine, but our sleds were in woeful condition. She drove to Canadian Tire and returned with two new GT racing sleds. They cost $50 apiece.

Assembling things like GTs greatly exceeds my virtually non-existent mechanical capabilities. Luckily for me, when Gord got to our house he offered to help. We sat on the kitchen floor and surrounded ourselves with a slew of sled parts. After 30 minutes of head-scratching and tinkering we managed to put together a pair of GTs that looked more or less like the ones on the covers of the boxes. We both felt that applying the decals would take more time than it was worth, so we skipped that step.

The last thing we needed to do was fasten a slender tow-rope to the front of each sled. The instruction sheets didn't offer any helpful hints as to what type of knot to tie. The company probably figured if you couldn't come up with an effective knot, either you still drank from a sippy cup or you were just too damn stupid to own one of their sleds. Unfortunately, Gord and I both happen to be severely knot-challenged. We can intubate, throw in chest tubes and do spinal taps, but knots? Fuggedaboutit. What do we look like, sailors?

I was seriously considering giving up when an ancient memory of a knot I learned in Cubs decades prior lumbered out from some forgotten corner of my brain. I hastily replicated it before the memory receded.

I looked over to see how Gord was making out. I guess he never attended Cubs. He had tied a hideous Spanish Inquisition-looking knot on his sled. He was staring down at the tangled mess despondently. I couldn't resist: "Avast matey! That's quite the Frankenknot you've created there!"

"You can say that again," he said. "Oh well, no one said it had to be pretty. Let's go tobogganing!"

It was an ideal afternoon for sledding – only minus 10 degrees Celsius, a cobalt sky and tons of fresh powder. Best of all, we had the entire hill to ourselves! No hot-dogging snowboarders attempting death-defying grinds and shreds. No snowmobilers paying homage to Saint Knievel. No tinnitus poster boys with portable boom boxes blasting out their favourite speed-metal arias for our listening pleasure *(Hey buddy, did it ever occur to you that maybe the rest of North America doesn't want to hear Napalm Death at 10 billion decibels?)*. Just two middle-aged guys and their kids. We had a great time.

Two hours later one of my daughters announced she needed to go to the bathroom. It was about time for supper anyway, so I told Gord we were going to head back home. He said he and the boys would go down the hill one last time and then meet us at our house. I gathered up as many of the sliding accessories as I could handle and walked home with the girls.

Gord and his boys arrived not long afterwards. We washed up and had supper. After supper the kids played games until they were exhausted. At bedtime Gord read them all a story. When the last child finally drifted off to sleep, Gord, Jan and I went to the kitchen and raided the fridge for beer and snacks. We stayed up chatting until midnight.

After breakfast the next morning we asked the kids what they wanted to do. Their answer was unanimous: sledding. Gord was the first to get his snowsuit on. He went outside to round up the gear but returned shortly afterwards with a quizzical look on his face.

"I found all the crazy carpets, but there's only one GT outside," he said. "Where's the other one?"

"Probably in the garage," I replied.

"No, I already checked in there. Do you remember where you left them when you got home last night?"

"Them? I only brought one back. Didn't you bring the second one? It was tied to that bench near the top of the hill."

"I must have walked right by it. I guess I figured you had taken both of them with you."

"Don't worry about it," I said. "It'll still be there. This is a friendly little town. It's not like anyone's going to rip off a GT."

The boys finished pulling on their boots and ran outside. My daughters weren't quite ready yet, so I told Gord to go on ahead. Five minutes later the girls and I departed.

When we emerged from the path that opens onto the clearing at the top of the hill I spotted Gord right away. It wasn't that difficult – at 6-foot-5 he was easily the tallest of the dozen or so people milling about. Even from a distance I could tell something was amiss. I waved at him and shouted, "Did you find it?"

Instead of answering, he loped over to me. *Uh-oh.*

"There was no GT tied to the bench," he whispered, "but that kid over there has one that looks exactly like ours." He jerked his thumb in the direction of the throng of people at the summit.

"Do you think it's ours?" I asked.

"I'm pretty sure."

"Did you talk to him?"

"Yeah."

"What did he say?"

"He said he got it for Christmas."

I went over to take a look.

The boy was facing the opposite direction as I approached. There was a GT immediately behind him. I scrutinized it closely. In addition to being brand spanking new and sticker-free, it was sporting the same abominable knot. How suspicious can you get? I tapped our suspect on the shoulder.

He twisted around lazily and appraised me. He was a gangly 12-year-old boy with saffron hair, an explosion of freckles and pale blue eyes. A hint of a smirk played about his mouth.

"Hi, I'm Dr. Gray," I said. "What's your name?"

"Josh."

"Josh, this GT looks a lot like the one I accidentally left out here last night. Do you think it could be mine?"

He tilted his head back, looked me straight in the eye and said, "Nope, it's mine."

"When did you get it?"

"At Christmas."

"Are you sure, Josh?"

"Yep." He turned away from me in a blatantly dismissive manner. I could feel my hackles rising.

"Hang on, Josh; I'm not quite finished yet. Like I said, I'm pretty sure this is my GT. What's your mother going to tell me if I call her and ask if you got a GT for Christmas?"

He wasn't expecting that. His smug look faltered.

"Um . . . ."

"What's your last name, Josh?"

"Uh . . . ." He started to fidget.

"What's your phone number? I've got a cell phone right here in my pocket." Of course I was bluffing, but he didn't know that. The last remnants of his cockiness vanished.

"I don't know!" he bleated nervously.

"Do you seriously expect me to believe you don't know your own phone number? Come on, Josh; give me a break. What's your phone number? Maybe I'll talk to your father, instead."

His eyes widened in horror.

"I promise you, I don't know!" he wailed.

By this time several curious snowboarders had coalesced around us. A few of them started snickering.

"I promise you, I don't know!" one of them trilled in a squeaky Josh-like voice. The rest of them guffawed loudly.

"Josh, this is my GT, isn't it?"

"Y-yes," he stammered at his boots.

"What's it called when you say things that aren't true?" Gord asked him pointedly.

"L-lying." I relieved him of his plunder and gave it to Kristen. She hopped on the sled and went rocketing down the hill. Josh slunk away guiltily.

An hour later I was sitting on the bench taking a breather when Josh approached me.

Aha, he's come back to apologize. There's hope for him yet!

"Dr. Gray?" he ventured, eyes downcast.

"Yes?"

"Can I borrow your GT?"

Legerdemain (*Sleight Of Hand*)

Most weekday mornings I do a couple of scheduled minor procedures in the emergency department. Patients used to have to sign a consent form prior to undergoing minor procedures, but a few years ago that antiquated ritual was laid to rest. If registering at the front desk, sitting in the waiting room for half an hour and then remaining perfectly still on an uncomfortable stretcher while being poked and prodded by sharp instruments isn't proof enough that consent has been given, I don't know what is.

Wart removals and cortisone injections are usually quick and predictable. Biopsies, on the other hand, are an entirely different kettle of fish. Minor biopsies involve removing only a tiny sliver of tissue, so sometimes the entire procedure lasts no longer than a few minutes. In those cases it probably takes more time to fill out the various forms that accompany the specimen to the laboratory than it does to remove the lesion itself. There are times, however, when much larger blocks of tissue need to be expunged. Sometimes this is because the lesion itself is bulky; other times it's because the mole looks cancerous and we want to make sure all traces of it are eliminated. When it comes to lumps-and-bumps removal, there's nothing more disconcerting than receiving a pathology report that states the lesion in question is an incompletely excised malignant melanoma.

When I enter the treatment room I always ask my patient to confirm the procedure they're expecting me to perform. I find this is the best way to avoid injecting the wrong joint, removing the wrong mole, etc. Why make malpractice lawyers' jobs any easier than they already are? After I've verified we're both on the same wavelength I begin to gather the necessary hardware. If my patient has that familiar white-knuckled look I'll chit-chat with them as I assemble the supplies. First I place my latex-free gloves on the counter behind me. I then open the biopsy tray and pile the scalpel, needles, syringes and suture material onto it.

Next I pour chlorhexidine into the stainless steel bowl. After instructing the patient to lie down, I adjust the spotlight to ensure the lesion is optimally illuminated. When I'm satisfied with the lighting I put on my disposable blue facemask. Breathing with the facemask on always makes my glasses fog up, so after a few seconds of looking like a total loser I dispense with the glasses and deposit them on the counter. I snap on my gloves with dramatic flourish, draw up the local anaesthetic and whirl like Zorro to face the doomed lesion (*okay, so maybe not quite like Zorro*). I wash the skin with the antiseptic solution and drape clean towels around the area to maintain a sterile surgical field. I give the patient fair warning that I'm about to start injecting, then infiltrate the vicinity with the anaesthetic. Once my target is fully frozen (does *this* hurt? – *poke, poke*) I'm ready to proceed.

I gently rest the blade of the scalpel on the surface of the skin. A moment later I apply firm downward pressure. As the blade bites into the tissue I begin carving an ellipse around the lesion. Sometimes bright red blood wells up through the incision, forcing me to stop and compress the area with a wad of gauze until it settles. Fresh blood has an unmistakable odour. I used to find it disturbing, but now some days I hardly even notice it. When the field is no longer obscured by blood I resume cutting a swath through epidermis, dermis and subcutaneous tissue. Once the ellipse is complete I fillet the chunk of flesh out and drop it into the specimen jar. Oftentimes I'll put a couple of dissolvable stitches deep inside the wound before closing the more superficial layers with regular suture. I dry the skin with some fresh gauze, slap on an adhesive dressing and *voila!* Mission Accomplished, as Dubya would say.

For most physicians, these basic procedures become automatic. Like driving a car, once the skill has been mastered we no longer need to devote every iota of our attention to the process every time we do it. For certain tasks it's safe to temporarily activate cruise control and give the overseeing, self-aware part of our brains a chance to disconnect and take a breather. Don't worry – it checks in regularly to monitor how things are going. It just doesn't strain to analyze and micromanage every nanosecond of the procedure. It's a useful little technique that helps stave off burnout.

Another tactic we often use to help us cope better is disengagement. We separate ourselves from some of the inherently distasteful things we're required to do every day by mentally stepping back and viewing our actions from a distance. I'm not sure whether the process is partially under conscious control or if it's completely subliminal, but either way it's a nifty trick. It doesn't work perfectly every time, though. Once in a while I'll be poised to begin a procedure when it will suddenly occur to me that my mind hasn't yet slid into its neutral "physician mode." In other words, the non-medical part of my cerebral cortex hasn't politely stepped aside to let the Vulcan take over. Worse yet, occasionally the veil lifts right when I'm smack dab in the middle of something. When this happens I become a doctor with John Q. Citizen's viewpoint. This has the effect of transiently turning my perspective on what I'm doing inside out, which can lead to some jarring observations. For example, when the biopsy scalpel I'm wielding punctures my patient's skin and rivulets of blood start to flow, every now and then I think *Holy crap! I just cut this guy with a scalpel! What's that all about?*

Sometimes this parallactic view makes me consider other procedures in my therapeutic repertoire in an entirely different light:

Rapid sequence intubations – I give critically ill patients drugs that completely paralyze every voluntary muscle in their body. I then glide a plastic ET tube past their inert vocal cords in order to manually take over the process of breathing for them. If I can't get the tube in, their risk of a bad outcome increases exponentially. *Zoinks!*

Chest tube insertion – I dissect the chest wall of a conscious person down to the level of the lining of the lungs, then thrust a tube the size of a garden hose into their pleural space in order to drain air, blood or pus. *Seriously?*

Neonatal resuscitation – I try to insufflate life into floppy, blue newborns. *Did I really sign up for this?*

Lumbar punctures – I slide a four-inch needle between two of the lower lumbar vertebrae in order to obtain a sample of cerebrospinal fluid for laboratory analysis. *Just think of it as the human equivalent of maple syrup tapping . . . .*

Central lines – I insert sasquatch-sized IVs into people's necks for better venous access. *Ack!*

Corneal foreign body removals – I use needles and spinning brushes to scrape fragments of metal and other embedded objects off the surface of patients' eyes. *Hold still now . . . .*

Assisting at laparotomies – I help the surgeon open someone up and exteriorize their guts for inspection and repair. *Are you kidding me?*

Prostate exams – I . . . whaaat? *Let's not even go there!*

Fortunately, these unexpected episodes of viewing things through non-medical eyes are so short-lived, they're almost stillborn. Their evanescent nature allows me to quickly return to the strange realm of Asclepius where things that would under normal circumstances be considered outrageous are, for now, perfectly acceptable. I believe this mental sleight of hand is one of the Jedi mind tricks that allow us to perform unpleasant procedures without becoming overwhelmed by them. I also suspect it may help prevent us from getting hopelessly mired in an endless loop of recursive thoughts.

But then again, what the hell do I know?

Sometimes the Voices Are Real . . . .

Last Tuesday my morning office went into double overtime. When it finally wrapped up I went to the hospital to see some inpatients. My rounds there finished at 1:25. My afternoon office was scheduled to begin at 1:30, so I decided to skip lunch. Unfortunately, within a minute of making that decision I was feeling so wretched I could hardly stand myself. For those of you who don't know me, just ask Jan - *nobody* does pathetic like I do. I hopped in my car and drove to Tim Hortons with visions of a chicken salad sandwich dancing in my head.

As I pulled onto the far end of the lot I happily noted there were no cars in the drive-through lane. What fabulous luck! I was cruising towards the microphone when suddenly Methuselah's older brother shuffled out from between two parked cars and directly into my path. I mashed on the brakes. He stopped and turned to peer at me through incredibly thick glasses. I waited for him to give some modest display of apology – a nod or wave or perhaps a sheepish half-smile. Instead he curled his lip harder than Billy Idol and continued on his way. By the time he finished creaking past, another car glided in from the opposite direction and stopped at the drive-through microphone. I pulled up behind it, gnashing my teeth and cursing Geritol under my breath. I briefly contemplated leaving, but I was too hungry. I decided to wait and see what they ordered. If it was something quick like coffee, I'd place an order. If not, I'd leave.

I snuck a look at the person in the vehicle in front of me and recognized her to be Mrs. Hatter, a tenuously-controlled schizophrenic. As usual, she was busy taking enormous drags from one of her supersized homemade cigarettes.

"Welcome to Tim Hortons! Can I take your order please?"

Mrs. Hatter looked straight up at the sky for a few seconds. She then cocked her head to the side like a pigeon and scanned the horizon in all directions. When she was satisfied all sectors were clear she resumed puffing.

"Uh, welcome to Tim Hortons . . . . Can I take your order please?" She did her sky inspection once again. This time she also checked the glove compartment, her purse and the back seat. She then stubbed out her cigarette and lit a new one.

My stomach grumbled loudly. I debated whether or not I should walk over to her and explain that *this* particular voice happened to be coming from the drive-through microphone. I ended up deciding to wait one more minute and hope she figured it out on her own. *Are you there, God? It's me, Donny. Help her figure it out, okay? And while you're at it, would you mind encouraging her to order just a coffee? Much obliged.*

"Hello? Anyone there? Would you like to place an order?"

"Yeah, I'm gonna take der chili deal an' a big coffee. An' maybe a couple of dem donuts. Hey, youse guys got any sandwiches? What kinda soups you sell 'ere, anyways? Anyting on special today? How much you tink dis is gonna cost?"

I burnt rubber out of the parking lot.

Status Interrupticus

Mr. Golding is a 50-year-old man with a strong family history of heart disease. His cholesterol is astronomical and dietary adjustments have failed miserably. I've called him in to get him started on a cholesterol-lowering medication.

"Hey doc!"

"Hi Mr. Golding."

"I guess my cholesterol's still pretty high, eh?"

"Yes, that's right."

"How high was it?"

"It was – "

"I just can't figure out why it won't come down, doc! For breakfast every morning I eat a small bowl of Corn Flakes with skimmed milk. After that I have an apple or an orange, or sometimes I'll take a glass of juice instead."

"That's good – "

"Real juice, mind you, not fake junk like Tang. I can't believe astronauts used to drink that stuff!"

"Can't say I've ever – "

"If I'm still hungry, I'll have toast with margarine. Is that Becel stuff any good?"

"What?"

"According to the ads on TV, it's really low in fat or something."

"Most dieticians say – "

"For lunch the wife fixes me a tuna sandwich. I must have told her a million times to go easy on the mayo, but she still slathers it on like crazy! Hey, doc, do you think she's trying to kill me? Har-har!"

"Let's hope not. Anyway, your cholesterol's still very high, so – "

"Oh, and supper! What we eat depends on what day of the week it is. Usually Monday's spaghetti night, but sometimes we have . . . doc? Where are you going? Doc?"

The Call of the Wild *(Sorry, Jack!)*

Last September I went on a canoe trip with four colleagues. I'm not much of a *voyageur*, but I figure if you live in northern Ontario you may as well get out and enjoy the great outdoors once in a while. Sometimes the wild north gets a little *too* wild, though . . . .

It was close to 4:00 on a chilly Wednesday afternoon by the time we finished cramming our supplies into the back of the truck. The drive from our town to Missinaibi Provincial Park was upwards of 400 kilometres, the last one-fifth of which involved slaloming down an unbelievably bumpy logging road.

When we were about 30 minutes from our destination a host of ominous-looking black clouds began boiling across the sky. By the time we arrived at the main entrance to the park it was raining torrentially. We're talking biblical here. Noah. The floating zoo. A Farewell to Unicorns. You get the picture. We scoured the grounds for a vacant campsite. At last we found a cramped spot with a multitude of rocks and tree roots protruding through the grass. Welcome to Trump Towers! We pitched our tents in the pouring rain, ate a cold supper and crawled into our sleeping bags. As I prepared to enter the Dreaming I tried not to think about the warm bed I had left behind.

The next morning was cool and overcast, but at least it wasn't raining. We broke camp and trooped down to the dock. The lake was steel grey. The small cove the dock jutted into was calm, but the rest of the lake looked choppy. As we loaded our provisions into the two canoes, a gnarled old Grizzly Adams look-alike hobbled over.

"Goin' out on the lake?" he queried.

"Yes, we have a four-day trip planned," I replied. "Can't wait to get started!"

"Dern cold out."

"You're right, it is a bit nippy."

"Ah've been out here more'n 25 years, an' you wouldn't catch me goin' out on a mornin' like this!"

"Oh. Well, according to the Weather Network – "

He pointed at the kayak I had borrowed for the trip.

"Which one of yehs planning on using that contraption?"

"I am. As a matter of fact, this will be my first trip in a kayak!" I declared proudly.

For a moment his rheumy eyes widened in disbelief. He then snorted derisively and stumped away. I could have sworn I heard him mutter something about "dern city fools" under his breath.

While the canoes launched I zipped up my water-resistant windbreaker, secured my life jacket and pushed the kayak into the lake. Although it was light and handled easily, I found it hard to keep up with the canoes. After several minutes of paddling we got out of the cove and into the main body of the lake. Out there the winds were much stronger and the water was rough. Our progress slowed to a crawl. I conjured up a mental image of our trip map. We had to paddle approximately half the length of the lake before we got to the origin of the Missinaibi River. At our current pace, that was going to take four or five hours. If we hugged the shoreline there would be much less wind to contend with, but we'd be adding a lot of extra mileage to the trip. I had no idea how to do that clever barrel-roll manoeuvre that allows you to remain seated and flip a capsized kayak right-side up, so if I ended up in the drink I'd have to swim for dry land. I was therefore hoping the canoeists would stick close to shore. Instead, they chose the low-mileage option and headed straight for the centre of the lake.

Kayak paddles have a nasty tendency to dribble water onto you with each stroke, so by the end of the first hour I was soaked. By the end of the second hour the canoes were two tiny dots bobbing on the horizon and I was starting to wonder what the hell I was doing out in the middle of a freezing-cold lake in a kayak. Right about then I mistimed one of my strokes and plunged the paddle deep into a trough instead of a crest. This brought my centre of gravity way outside the kayak, which caused it to tilt nearly 90 degrees sideways. I spent the next two or three eternities staring down into the churning water and wishing I owned a caul as my vessel teetered on the verge of rolling over. It then made a loud grinding noise and shuddered back to its normal axis. After that I quit daydreaming.

An hour later we stopped at an island to rest. I was completely drenched. While I wrung out my clothes and poured lake water out of my ducky boots, my friend Will passed some mugs of soup around.

"Th-th-th-thanks!" I stammered. My teeth were chattering so badly it's a wonder I didn't bite my tongue off. The soup was piping hot and it warmed us up quickly. Before long we were back in the water, full of enthusiasm and ready for anything.

By the time we entered the Missinaibi River the wind had died down considerably. We put ashore for a planning conference. According to our trip map, Quittagene Rapids was just around the bend. Although it was listed as only a Class II rapid (Class VI being Niagara Falls), the notes warned it became trickier and more technical when water levels were intermediate. We scouted it out, took an informal vote and decided to try running it. Will and Larry volunteered to go first. They started off promisingly, but a short while later they spun out in an eddy and ended up facing backwards. Unless you're Super Dave Osborne, going back asswards through rapids is highly discouraged. They wisely abandoned the attempt and returned to the riverbank. From there they used the canoe's painter ropes to manually guide it safely through the foaming whitewater.

I was considering doing the same thing with my kayak when Yves winked at me and said: "Chance of a lifetime, man! You can do it!" Of course I had to take the challenge. We men are kind of stupid that way. Fortunately for me, it wasn't as terrifying as it looked – the kayak seemed to naturally seek out the less riotous channels, so all I had to do was provide a little muscle and take evasive action whenever it looked like I was about to have a close encounter with a pointy rock. Ducking to avoid the overhanging sweepers and blasting out between the final set of boulders at the bottom was a real rush! A few minutes later the second canoe made its way through. We paddled for another hour before calling it quits and setting up camp for the night.

The next morning dawned cold. A beautiful ghost-like mist cloaked the river. Eventually the sun rose high enough to burn the haze away. We ate breakfast, packed up and slid our vessels into the water. The wind was at our backs and we had no major portages that day, so we made excellent time. By early evening we arrived at our new campsite. We pitched the tents, started a fire and ate a hearty supper. That night a thousand stars filled the heavens.

Saturday was our designated rest day. Activities included reading, writing, swimming, hiking, bird-watching and fishing. After lunch Will and John decided to paddle 30 minutes downstream to recon Sun Rapids. It was listed as a Class II technical, so they figured they wouldn't have any trouble running it in an empty canoe. Several hours later they were still missing in action and the rest of us were beginning to worry. We were just getting ready to go search for them when they paddled into view. They were sodden and their canoe was sporting an impressive array of fresh dings and scrapes. It turned out they had run the rapids twice.

The first time they selected a route that had them pass to the right of a huge boulder in the middle of the whitewater. The second time around they attempted to pass the boulder on the left, but the current caught them broadside and slammed them against it. At the moment of impact they were both catapulted into the turbulence and their paddles floated away. The incredible force of the rushing water pinned the canoe in place and bent it into a U-shape, inside-out, around the rock. Amazingly, it didn't snap in two. While Will swam downstream through the rapids to retrieve the paddles, John stood in the pounding, chin-high water and struggled to pry the canoe loose. It had taken a unique combination of prayers, curses and Herculean effort, but eventually they were successful in both finding the paddles and freeing the canoe. Thanks to the Royalex material the canoe was made of, it sprang back into its normal shape as soon as it was off the rock. The journey back to our site depleted whatever little energy John and Will had left. They both slept like logs that night.

The next day we were all careful to give due respect to Sun Rapids' now infamous canoe-eating boulder. It wasn't difficult to spot, given the fact it was the only rock in the river with a wide strip of red paint on it. While the others lined the canoes down river left, I cautiously navigated my vessel through a kayak-friendly channel. The ensuing Barrel Rapids was also handled with kid gloves.

At last we arrived at the marshes of Peterbell, home to a wide variety of northern Ontario flora and fauna and the border of the Chapleau Crown Game Preserve. Years ago Peterbell was a thriving logging outpost community, but now it is completely devoid of human inhabitants. A VIA Rail train passes through it three times a week, and if a canoe party is waiting by the tracks the train stops and picks them up. We dragged our provisions ashore and set up camp in a field. Our plan was to get up early the next day and schlep our stuff to the tracks. When the train made its scheduled mid-morning appearance we'd be home free. We got a good blaze going, ate supper under a molten sky and traded war stories about prior canoe trips.

At 10:30 that night, Larry, Will and John turned in. Yves and I were still wide awake, so we stayed up late kibitzing. Shortly after 11:00 Yves stepped beyond the perimeter of flickering light cast by the fire to empty his bladder. A minute later he was back.

"I just saw a dog," he said.

"Yves, we're at least a hundred klicks away from the nearest house. Are you sure it was a dog?"

"Uh-huh. I think I'll go call it. Maybe it's hungry!"

Before I could say another word he turned around and was engulfed by the darkness once again.

"Here, doggy, doggy! Here, boy! Here .... *Sacré bleu!*"

In an instant he was back beside me. He looked totally freaked.

"What?" I asked.

"That was no dog!"

"What was it?"

"A wolf!"

"Yikes!"

We put another armful of dry logs on the fire and stayed up an extra hour before retiring to our sleeping bags.

At 0-dark-30 hours I was awakened by the sound of Larry climbing back into our two-man tent after the traditional early morning if-I-hold-it-any-longer-I'll-explode pee.

"Hey," I mumbled groggily, "While you were out there, did you happen to see that wolf?"

"What wolf?"

Just then a piercing, high-pitched howl began. It was so loud, it sounded like it was coming from the outside flap of our tent. Larry's eyes nearly bulged out of his head.

"What the hell is that?" he whispered.

"A wolf. Yves saw it last night."

The howling stopped abruptly. The sudden silence was almost as jarring as the unexpected wolf call had been.

"Should we –?"

The howling began again, except this time it was eight times louder because many new voices were participating. The blood-curdling, ululating chorus went on and on, from every possible direction. Then it ceased, leaving echoes ricocheting around the insides of our skulls.

My heart was jack-hammering in my chest. Talk about a dramatic wakeup call! If those critters were hungry, our thin polyester tents weren't going to be much of a deterrent to them. We armed ourselves with flashlights and unzipped the tent flap.

Yves, Will and John spilled out of their tent just as Larry and I emerged from ours. It was still dark enough to prevent us from seeing much past the glowing embers in the fire pit. Larry flicked on his flashlight and cast a beam of light northward into the gloom. A pair of green wolf eyes stared back at him. He aimed his flashlight south. Another wolf. East, west and several ordinal points in between – you guessed it. We were surrounded by a wolf pack.

"Say, guys," I said, hoping no one noticed my voice's sudden ascent to castrato. "Do wolves ever, um, *eat* people?"

"I . . . don't think so," replied Will.

"Are you sure about that?"

"No."

The wolves stared at us silently for a long time before melting away into the shadows.

Not surprisingly, no one wandered off by themselves to wash their face in the river that morning. Instead, we skipped breakfast, set a new world record for disassembling a campsite and double-timed it to the train tracks. We were all very happy campers when the VIA train finally appeared in the distance.

Can't wait for next year's trip!

Tabula Rasa

Could someone please remind me why we strive so hard to keep Harry alive?

Harry is a severely handicapped middle-aged man. Cauliflower-shaped tumours burst out of his scalp and protrude through his patchy hair at irregular intervals. He grinds his teeth incessantly. It's a loud, grating noise that makes you want to scream.

He has no intelligible speech. To be honest, he has nothing even vaguely resembling any sort of communication. He is unable to use his limbs in any purposeful manner, so he is permanently diapered and confined to a wheelchair.

Despite his group home attendants' best efforts to feed him carefully, he still has frequent episodes of food aspiration and chest infections that leave him wheezing and gasping for air. Whenever this happens he is immediately brought to our emergency department for treatment. We dutifully admit him to the medical ward and start him on oxygen, suctioning, bronchodilator inhalations and intravenous antibiotics. Sometimes he becomes so ill we have to intubate him and put him on a ventilator.

He has some relatives who have power of attorney over his affairs. They live less than an hour away. In the nine years I've known Harry they haven't visited him once. I've called them on two occasions to ask whether they'd consider switching his code status to "do not resuscitate." Both times their answer was the same: "Keep him alive, doc – we've been thinking about coming up to see him sometime."

So the battle to save Harry continues. Day after day I go into his room and watch him struggle to breathe. It's a Greek epic being played out in a hospital bed; an endless tragedy with a cast of one, viewed by an audience of one. To me, Harry embodies the combined suffering of Prometheus, Tantalus and Orpheus. Sir Laurence himself couldn't evoke such pathos.

He cranes his head to the side in an attempt to look at me whenever I place my stethoscope on his misshapen chest. His moist, cow-like eyes roll in all directions. I often wonder if he's going to bite me. It's an irrational thought; Harry is wholly incapable of aggression.

Does Harry have thoughts? If so, how does he perceive this world? Is it a magical place or an unending horror? Are we his saviours or his tormentors? Does he admire us or despise us? Does he hope for life or death?

It may well be that his mind is a blank slate. If that's the case, perhaps we shouldn't stand in his way the next time we see him lumbering towards the brink.

Some Patients Are Never Ready

Two years ago Max noticed a trace of blood in his stool. Colonoscopy revealed bowel cancer. Staging investigations didn't show any evidence of tumour spread. It was felt he had a good chance of surgical cure, so arrangements were made for a bowel resection.

The surgery went well. To everyone's relief, the sampled lymph nodes came back negative for cancer cells. In the weeks following the operation it became evident that his surgeon and his oncologist held opposing views regarding the potential benefits of adjunctive chemo. After carefully considering both options, Max declined chemotherapy.

Six months later I was in the radiology suite looking at a surveillance x-ray of Max's chest when I noticed a small lesion near the apex of his right lung. *Uh-oh. Hard times ahead.*

"What does it mean?" he asked when I saw him in my office the following day. "The cancer hasn't come back, has it?"

"I hope not, but it's possible," I answered evasively. "I'm going to send you back to the cancer clinic. They'll run some more tests and then do a biopsy."

The scans confirmed our worst fear – the spot on his lung looked cancerous. No other traces of malignancy were found, though. The chest surgeon was hopeful the lesion was a new primary rather than a metastasis. If it had arisen *de novo*, removing it could be curative. If it turned out to be a metastatic subsidiary of the original cancer, his long-term prognosis would be abysmal.

Max's lung surgery was uneventful. A month later he was back in my office to review his pathology results.

"Did they get it all?"

"It looks that way, judging by the reports."

"Was it related to the first cancer, or was this one brand new?" His voice quavered slightly.

"They're not sure – the pathology findings were inconclusive."

"How could I have gotten lung cancer, doc? I never smoked a day in my life!"

"Well, every once in a while a non-smoker gets lung cancer. Just bad luck, I guess."

"What happens next?"

"Chemotherapy."

The chemo left Max weak and hairless, but he didn't care. Anything to reduce the chances of a recurrence.

Six months later an abdominal ultrasound picked up a new lesion on his liver. Max nearly cried when I told him.

"What do we do now?" he asked. I sent him back to the cancer treatment centre. The chemo regimen he was given failed. So did the next one. After the third failure I tried to gently broach the topic of terminal cancer and palliative care, but he recoiled. "I don't want to know how long I've got. I'm not ready to die yet."

Max has undergone many more chemo and radiation treatments. Each successive scan shows more lesions than the one before.

My patient now weighs about 90 pounds. We've run out of treatments to offer. Although his emaciated body is riddled with cancer and his candle is slowly guttering, he's still not yet ready to talk about dying.

I don't think he ever will be.

Shotgun Bubba

"My husband and I are worried about Bubba. He's been acting really weird lately and we think his schizophrenia might be getting out of control. He's got this idea there are people hiding in the attic and they're plotting to kill him."

"Gee, that's too bad. We may have to increase his antipsychotic medication."

"Thanks, doc. Things have gotten so out of hand Bubba's even refusing to go outside because he's worried he'll get kidnapped."

"That sounds pretty paranoid. Is he saying or doing anything that makes you feel nervous or unsafe in any way?"

"No, nothing like that."

"Are you sure?"

"Well, come to think of it, a couple of nights ago I was sitting on the toilet in the middle of the night when all of a sudden the bathroom door banged open and there he was with a shotgun in his hands!"

"A *shotgun?*"

"Yeah."

"Was it *loaded?*"

"Oh yes, we always keep our guns loaded. Sometimes we get bears on our property."

"Good grief!"

"Since then he's taken to walking around the house with the shotgun all the time. He says he's seeing spooky faces in the windows and holding a gun makes him feel safer."

"Your paranoid, psychotic and hallucinating brother is patrolling your house night and day with a loaded shotgun and that doesn't worry you?"

"Why should we worry? He never points it at us."

Disneyfied

Little Tiffany's dad has brought her in for her four-month well-baby check. She's been healthy and so far everything looks normal. While I'm examining her eyes I ask her father: "Do you have any concerns about her vision?"

"No doc, as far as we know, her eyes are fine."

"That's good," I reply.

"And she sure loves her Disney!"

"What?"

"Disney movies, doc. The cartoon ones! She just loves them!"

"She watches Disney movies?"

"Yeah, she can't get enough of them!"

"But she's only four months old! How long has she been watching television?"

"Oh, since she was about a month and a half. We put the TV right up beside her crib and prop her up on a pillow. Sometimes she'll watch an entire movie! You should see her smile!"

"Um, several studies have suggested it's better for kids to not watch television until they're at least a year old."

"Those guys don't know what they're talking about."

Slippage

Things are slipping. It's a steady, relentless process. Every day another inappropriate behaviour crawls out from under a rock and suns itself in plain view. What's going on? And where will it end?

Not that long ago even the snarkiest adolescent would at least have made a token effort to not swear within earshot of an adult. My, how times have changed. Some of the language you hear from kids nowadays is harsh enough to make your ears bleed. More than once I've had to hastily round up my children and flee a playground in order to escape the profane chatter exploding all around us. I'm not just talking about the odd expletive being lobbed around. That doesn't even make me *blink* anymore. No, I'm talking about the air being saturated with verbal shrapnel from continuous f-bombing. It's like a sonic blitzkrieg. I'm no choirboy, but I've got my limits.

Where are kids learning such extreme language? Everywhere. Reality television, ultraviolent video games, laxly-censored movies, gangsta rap, shock radio . . . . The vulgarity envelope gets pushed a little further every day. You don't have to be a nuclear physicist to recognize the linear relationship between unsupervised access to certain media and Potty Mouth Syndrome.

To make matters worse, there doesn't appear to be a lower age limit to this worrisome phenomenon. Last fall Ellen started grade four. One day she was helping out in a kindergarten classroom at lunchtime. One of the littluns she was in charge of made a mess and casually strolled away from it. When Ellen reminded him to clean up, he glared at her and told her to f**k off. What's next, fetuses cursing in utero?

Generation Z also seems to have no qualms about littering. It's hard to believe the amount of garbage strewn around some playgrounds and schoolyards. The same can be said about the routes along which kids walk to get to school. The elderly widow across the street from us allows neighbourhood kids to cut through her yard on their way to and from school. How is her kindness repaid? Every day her property gets littered with empty pop cans and junk food debris. I'm surprised she doesn't complain. Maybe she's afraid to.

Our daughters get frustrated whenever they see people litter. Once Alanna asked a classmate why he dumps his trash on the playground every recess. His reply? "Someone else will pick it up." I shouldn't demonize kids who litter, though. Children learn through instruction and observation. A few months ago I went to the washroom at a movie theatre. A little boy and his father were standing in front of the urinals. The boy was holding a Kleenex. Try as he might, he just couldn't manage to unzip his pants while maintaining his grip on the tissue paper. Eventually he asked his dad for help. "Just drop it on the floor," his father advised. The boy complied. It was still on the floor when they left.

Recently I was waiting for a bus in Toronto when a pack of preteen girls carrying bags of McFood emerged from the subway. They leaned against a nearby retaining wall and proceeded to wolf down their pink-slime burgers. Despite the presence of a large garbage can a few feet away they all threw their leftover food, condiments and cups on the sidewalk. Partway through their feast the city worker responsible for keeping the area clean came by and swept up the mess. As soon as he was out of sight they tossed the rest of their garbage on the sidewalk and howled with laughter.

Yesterday I was out running when I came across an ice cream bar wrapper on the sidewalk. There were still flecks of unmelted ice cream on it, so I figured it must have been discarded only moments before. Half a block ahead of me a 12-year-old boy was pushing his bicycle up a hill. I jogged over to him and asked: "Did you just eat an ice cream bar?"

"Uh-huh."

"Is that the wrapper back there on the sidewalk?"

"Yeah."

"You shouldn't throw your garbage on the ground. That's called pollution, and it's bad for our community."

He thought about it for a second and then grinned.

"Okay." He rode back to the wrapper and put it in his pocket.

Perhaps there's hope for the future after all.

My Organic Patient

I'm back in the emergency department, my home away from home. *Run, rabbit, run . . . .*

Mrs. Organic and her 14-year-old daughter are waiting to see me in cubicle B. Organic Jr. has a suspicious-looking mole they'd like to have looked at. It's black, irregular and raised. Lately it's gotten a bit bigger.

"Well, I think this mole needs to be removed. It's a little too busy for me to do it right now, but if you like I can take it off tomorrow afternoon."

"How is that done?" O.J. inquires.

"I inject some local anaesthetic, remove the mole with a scalpel and then sew up the skin."

"How is the anaesthetic developed?"

"What?"

"How is the local anaesthetic manufactured? Do they use any live animals in the testing of it?"

"Our little Organic Jr. is very much against anything that's bad for the environment and endangered ecosystems," her mom pipes up. She's practically glowing with pride.

"I have no idea how it's manufactured."

"Do you think maybe I could have the procedure done without any freezing?" O.J. asks hopefully.

As long as you don't wiggle around and scream too much! Your Birkenstocks might fall off!

"I wouldn't really recommend that – it would be quite painful for you."

"I think I'll research it on the Internet and then decide."

"That sounds like a great idea! I'll await your call!"

The Wonderful World of Golf

Today my golf game was more frightening than *The Exorcist*. Anyone following me around with a movie camera would have had an instant horror classic on their hands. Divots the size of meteorites. Drives that dribbled to a halt less than 10 feet away. Missed putts any fetus could have sunk. Bizarre sideways shots that defied all known laws of physics. And let's not forget those complete whiffs that left me looking like The Incredible Human Pretzel. I was so pitiful, even the blackflies stayed away from me. It didn't always used to be this way. Believe it or not, I coulda been a contender. This is my sad tale.

I used to shake my head at golfers and their harebrained marches down the fairway. Who in their right mind would voluntarily spend hours of prime time chasing an irrelevant little dimpled ball all over hell's half acre? Obsessive nutbars, that's who. "Get a life!" I'd feel like yelling every time I passed a platoon of fanatics in Bermuda shorts traipsing around a golf course.

Near the end of my first year in medical school some of my classmates decided they were going to learn how to golf. They invited me to join them. Naturally, I declined. "A group of golfing doctors?" I scoffed. "How cliché can you get? Thanks, but no thanks." Over the years many more invitations came my way, but I avoided them all like the plague.

Last summer my sister-in-law and her husband somehow managed to coerce me into playing a round of golf with them. As I prepared to tee off on the first hole I remember thinking, "This is going to be brutal." It wasn't. By the end of the game I was golf's newest convert. I began hanging out at the local driving range. Within a month I was cranking out fairly consistent 200 yard drives. True, they were often directionally challenged, but let's not quibble over details, okay? I bought a set of clubs and started playing regularly. To my surprise, I wasn't half bad! My drives, chips, sand work and putts, though rough and unpolished, were respectable enough for a newb. Several regulars commented that my game had Potential. Delusions of future Tigerhood filled my head.

In October, cold weather terminated our short northern golf season. I put my clubs away reluctantly. "Next year will be awesome," I told myself.

Come the spring my game picked up right where it had left off. Each outing was a little better than the one before. One evening I arrived at the course with hopes of getting a few holes in before dusk. I was preparing to tee off when a voice behind me said, "Mind if I join you?"

I turned around to see one of my patients.

"Certainly," I replied.

My drive went 180 yards. His topped 300. I was impressed. We hopped into his cart and zoomed down the fairway. At the end of the first hole my score was six and his was three.

He led off on the second hole with another towering 300-yard blast. As I set my ball on the tee he said, "Would you care for some advice?"

"Sure!" Any tips from a player of his stature could only serve to strengthen my game, right?

"Well, first of all, don't bend your knees so much. And try to keep your left elbow straight when you make contact with the ball. Also, make sure you keep your head down – you tend to look up to see where the ball went. Another thing I've noticed is . . . ."

I struggled to incorporate his myriad suggestions into my swing. The end result was that by the time darkness fell I couldn't even hit the ball.

That was three months ago. I'm still trying to unlearn the tips that vaporized my fledgling game that fateful evening. Welcome to the wonderful world of golf. *Fore!*

Oops!

Yesterday evening I was playing ping-pong with my daughters when the telephone rang.

"Hello?"

"Hi Dr. Gray. This is Trish on unit 4. I know you're not on call, but Mr. Arcularis just died and you had asked to be notified when that happened."

"Thanks, Trish. I'll be there in a few minutes."

I drove to the hospital, retrieved my stethoscope from my locker and walked over to the ward. Halfway down the hall I met one of our new medical students.

"Zhora, do you know which room my patient who just died is in?"

"Room 10, I think."

"Thanks."

I opened the door to room 10 and stepped inside. A dozen teary-eyed people twisted around and stared at me. I didn't recognize any of them. Someone in a white lab coat was leaning over an inert figure in the bed. As I drew closer I realized it was the on-call physician. He appeared to be in the process of pronouncing a patient dead. A female patient. He looked befuddled when he saw me.

"Oh, I'm sorry Donovan," he said. "Was she your patient?" Then it hit me. *Two people died at the same time, and I'm in the wrong room!*

The mourners were practically staring a hole in me. They probably all thought I had arrived to make some sort of earth-shattering announcement. Why else would I be barging in on such an incredibly private moment? I wanted to withdraw unobtrusively, but I knew that if I back-pedalled out the door I'd look like a complete idiot. I therefore strode up to my colleague, cupped my hand to his ear and whispered: "I'm in the wrong room! Act like I'm telling you something important!"

"Ah, yes, I'll look into that right away!" he blurted. "Absolutely! One hundred percent!" He nodded sagely and stroked his chin a few times for added effect. It was a Razzie-worthy performance.

I mumbled a quick thank you, turned around and scuttled away. How embarrassing!

Cancer

Cancer is greedy. It starts off as a single cell that is different from the rest. It multiplies continuously, with absolute disregard for the inhibitory signals sent to it by neighbouring cells.

As it grows it compresses and invades adjacent structures with impunity. It sends emissaries via the blood vessels and lymphatics to remote locations within the body. Some of them find fertile ground and start new colonies of destruction. The malignancy relentlessly devours nutrients intended for normal cells. In the absence of timely medical intervention and a bit of luck, the host eventually withers and dies. Ironically, when that happens the cancer dies too. Death is the ultimate chemotherapy.

Most people with cancer would be more than willing to strike a deal with their tumour whereby the two would live symbiotically and share all available nutrients. Unfortunately, cancer has no interest in abiding by covenants. Its only desire is to grow. As a result, it grows until it kills the very organism that it needs to survive. Cancer isn't just greedy; it's stupid as well.

Recently a friend of mine died of cancer. They won't be making any feel-good movies about her demise anytime soon. Her death was not poignant and meaningful. It was ugly, protracted and pointless. She suffered tremendously. She fought hard, but as the seasons passed her independence gradually dissolved away.

As each therapeutic regimen failed her hope for a cure diminished, until one day it was gone. She became glassy-eyed and monosyllabic. She stopped eating and drinking. Eventually she lapsed into a coma. Her loyal family kept a grim bedside vigil.

On the morning she died, the emotional dam finally burst. A flood of tears of bitterness, sorrow and relief was released. The healing process began.

Betcha Can't Eat Just One

Buster is a 55-year-old hypertensive diabetic who brings new meaning to the term non-compliant. He takes his medications randomly, eats tons of junk, thumbs his nose at exercise and smokes a couple of packs a day.

Recently he had a heart attack that was complicated by a mild case of congestive heart failure. I treated him with the usual meds and admitted him to unit 4.

When I did rounds later that evening I found him happily munching away on a jumbo-sized bag of salt and vinegar chips.

"Buster, what are you doing eating chips?" I squawked. "You're supposed to be on a low-salt diet!"

"Oops, sorry, doc." He put them away sheepishly.

The next day I returned to see my star patient. To my astonishment he was in the process of finishing off another ginormous bag of chips.

"Buster, didn't I tell you yesterday to stay away from chips?

There's too much salt in them!"

"Relax, doc," he replied. "These are barbeque!"

Curious George

Last patient of the day at the office. What final malady awaits me on the other side of this closed door? Right now I've got about as much energy as a fading boxer in the clinch, so I'm hoping to close out with a no-brainer like a blood pressure check. I lift the chart out of the rack. To my dismay there are two more files hiding behind it. It's the three-for-one Family Special. I've been had! I open the door and step inside.

Mrs. Fregoli is frowning as she weighs herself. When she steps off the scale it creaks with relief. Six-year-old Rachael is perched on the edge of the examining table. She quickly scans the pockets of my lab coat to ensure that I'm not trying to smuggle any needles into the room. Her five-year-old brother George is playing with the framed photograph of my daughters on my desk. I relieve him of his newfound swag and secure it on a high shelf.

"Hi Mrs. Fregoli. How can I help you today?"

"Doctor, I think sometimes my heart goes lub-*lub* instead of lub-*dub*."

"Okay, I'll have a listen in a minute. And what's wrong with your children?"

"Oh, they're fine, but I figured since I was coming in to see you I might as well bring them along for checkups."

"All right, then." I turn to her daughter. "Hullo, Rachael. Is it okay if I look at you first?"

"Sure," she replies gamely.

I'm reaching for the wall-mounted otoscope when I realize George is rifling through one of the drawers of my supplies cabinet. His mother doesn't appear to be particularly perturbed by this.

"Stay out of those drawers please, George," I call to him. He races over to the door and starts yanking on the handle.

"No, Georgie," his mother says. He pulls a face and bunny-hops back to his chair.

Whoa, I bet he's a real handful.

I resume examining Rachael. I'm squinting down her left ear canal when a loud crash startles us both. George has somehow managed to knock several textbooks off my desk. He flashes us all an impish grin and pirouettes over to the sink.

"Don't touch that, Georgie," pleads his mother.

He turns both faucets on full blast and claps his hands in the torrent of water. Everything within a two-foot radius of the sink gets soaked. I turn off the taps, clean up the mess and gently steer him back to his seat. He sits still for a microsecond, then starts rocking from side to side. I return to Rachael's examination.

A minute later Mrs. Fregoli sighs heavily and says: "Would you believe my little Georgie just got a three-day suspension from kindergarten?"

What's not to believe?

"Why was he suspended?" I ask politely.

"Supposedly for poor behaviour. They say that instead of listening to his teacher, he just runs all over the place."

Sort of like he's doing right now?

George is merrily tearing around the room. He's pushing the three-wheeled stool I usually sit on. Every so often he bashes it into one of the walls.

BLAM!

"George, honey; please stop that. Like I was saying, doctor . . ."

BLAM!

I separate George from the stool. He stamps his feet and sits on the floor.

". . . I don't know what they're talking about. He's *never* any trouble at home," she finishes.

"Is this how his teachers say he behaves at school?" I ask, looking up at the flickering overhead lights. George is treating us all to a funky disco strobe light effect by rapidly oscillating the light switch.

"George, dear; please stop that. No doctor, apparently it's much worse than this. They say at school he's completely out of control. My husband and I think they must be exaggerating."

George is seriously overloading my occipital cortex with his pyrotechnic light show. *I can smell burnt toast!* Before my impending seizure erupts, I pry his moist little fingers off the switch.

"Stop that," I hiss at him through gritted teeth. He scowls at me and launches into some mutant cross between jumping jacks and burpees.

"They've been after me to get him tested for hyperactivity," his mum volunteers.

"Well, he certainly is exhibiting – "

"They also think he might have something called ODD, whatever that is," she continues.

"Oppositional Defiant Disorder," I explain.

"Huh?"

"ODD is an acronym for Oppositional Defiant Disorder."

"Whatever. Anyway, they've been trying to get our permission to have him tested for ADD as well as this ODD thing, but we told them to forget it."

George tips over the wastepaper basket.

"Why don't you want him tested?" I ask.

George is standing on the three-wheeled stool.

"Because there's nothing wrong with him," she replies.

Now he's doing the Macarena on the stool.

"Then why do you think he behaves like this?"

She looks at me like I'm denser than a neutron star.

"Isn't it obvious?" she asks incredulously.

I shake my head to indicate it's not.

"He's just curious!" she explains.

Curious George falls off the stool and lands on his butt.

"Ow, Mommy! That hurt!"

"Oh, my poor baby! Come let Mommy give you a big hug, Georgie!"

I'll probably get a letter from some flesh-eating personal injury litigation lawyer next week.

Cerumen

Last Sunday afternoon the populace stormed the ramparts and our ER was overrun by an army of bellyaches, chest pain, asthma, migraines, fever and minor trauma. Every time I turned around the receptionist was in dumping a fresh batch of charts on the desk. *Sorry*, she'd smile at me apologetically before hurrying back to her battle station. Even though I knew it wasn't her fault, I was beginning to dislike her anyway. Crappy days make me a tad irrational sometimes.

Four hours into the carnage the triage nurse handed me a chart and asked, "Would you mind seeing him next?"

"Sure," I replied. "Where is he?"

"In the third cubicle."

"What's wrong with him?"

"Earwax."

"Earwax?"

"Yep."

"Geez."

Allow me to explain. Ever since I was a little kid I've had this thing about earwax. Simply put, I don't like it. I don't even like my own earwax, let alone someone else's. The less earwax I see, the better. My other beef with earwax is that as far as acute-care medicine is concerned, impacted earwax is without a doubt the world's biggest non-emergency, particularly when the department is under siege.

I marched over to cubicle C with an electron cloud of negative thoughts whizzing around my head: Isn't this supposed to be an *emergency* department? Did this guy even *try* to book an office appointment with his family doctor? By the time I got there I had worked myself into quite a lather. I yanked back the partially drawn curtain and unleashed an intimidating glare. The gnomish 80-year-old man sitting on the stretcher blinked back at me in surprise. Then he smiled widely and said: "Hello, doctor! Sorry to be such a bother. I know you're terribly busy today." All of a sudden my petulance atomized. It's hard to be mad at someone who reminds you of your dear old great-grandfather.

"Hi Mr. Magoo. I'm Dr. Gray. How can I help you?"

"I have a lot of, um . . . ." He pointed to his left ear.

"Earwax?" I offered clairvoyantly.

"Yes, earwax! Do you have time to flush it out for me?"

"No problem, sir. I'll look after that right away."

I foraged the department for the appropriate hardware and returned to his cubicle. First I examined his ear with an otoscope to make sure his self-diagnosis was correct. His left ear canal was indeed chock-full of the stuff. It was Earwax Heaven in there – the legendary mother lode. Next I draped a thick towel around his neck and got him to hold a kidney basin under his left ear. I then went to the sink and filled a large, stainless-steel syringe with warm water.

"I'm going to flush your ear out now," I informed him. "It'll probably feel a little uncomfortable, but if there's any sharp pain please let me know right away, okay?" He nodded assent. I squirted a jet of water into his left ear canal. The fluid that drained back out was completely devoid of earwax. As I turned to refill the syringe with water, I noticed him stealthily inspecting the contents of the basin. I flushed again. Crystal-clear returns. You could have used the water in the basin for an Evian ad. I motioned for him to pass it to me so I could empty it into the sink. Before handing it over he peered into it again and sighed.

"No wax," he said, his voice heavy with disappointment. I felt like I had struck out with the bases loaded. *Call me Casey. Some years ago – never mind how long precisely – having little or no money in my purse . . . .*

"Don't worry sir, we're not finished yet," I reassured him hastily as I dumped the water down the drain. I refilled the syringe with fresh water and tried again. This time there were a few specks of wax in the effluent. When he caught sight of them, his eyes widened.

"Look!" he said excitedly. "Look!"

"What?"

"Wax!"

"That's nice."

I repositioned the basin under his ear and flushed one more time. A brownish glob shot out of his ear canal. It looked big enough to be a vital organ.

"Look! Look!" he said, waving the basin around a couple of millimetres away from my nose. Some of the fluid sloshed out onto my lab coat. "A chunk! A chunk!" He was practically yodeling. I hazarded a glance. A huge, turd-like piece of earwax was half-submerged in the now-sludgy water. "I can hear!" he shouted. He deposited the basin on the counter, doffed the towel and shook my hand. "Thank you, doctor!" And with that, he was gone; one helluva satisfied customer. I sat on the stretcher with the intention of taking a 20-second Zen break before rejoining the fray and had an unexpected Damascene conversion. That took all of what, three minutes? How often are we modern-day physicians presented with the opportunity to make a patient *that* happy with such a quick, inexpensive, low-tech procedure?

So now I try really hard not to *kvetch* too much whenever someone presents to my ER requesting ear syringing. But I do have to confess – I'm still not that crazy about earwax.

For Better or Worse

I have a real love/hate relationship with my job. Some days I think being a doctor is the best job in the world. Why? Easy:

- It allows me to help people
- It's exciting
- It's intellectually stimulating
- It pays well

Other days I'm convinced practicing medicine is without a doubt the worst job *ever*. Why? Once again, easy:

- It's stressful
- It invades my personal life
- It burdens me with an absurd amount of responsibility
- It exposes me to a never-ending stream of demands from the public

Most days I'd never consider doing anything but medicine for a living, but there have certainly been times I've sworn I'd sooner dive head-first into a wood chipper than work one more shift in the ER.

One day recently my feelings regarding medicine went from one extreme to the other within a span of 30 minutes. Here's how it happened.

As is often the case on Wednesday mornings, by 10:30 the ER was completely gridlocked. When a cubicle finally became available, the nursing supervisor went out to get my next patient. To my dismay, she returned with Blair Neanderthal.

Blair is the president of our local Society for the Advancement of Alehouse Brawling. His abrasive personality is legendary. Unfortunately for me, this knuckle-dragging troglodyte also happens to be my patient. I hadn't seen him in more than a year, which made me wonder if he hadn't just completed yet another "timeout" in the slammer.

I reviewed the triage nurse's note. "Dental infection." Seemed fairly uncomplicated. I stepped into his cubicle and just about bounced off the force field of hostility crackling around him.

"I've been waiting for over an hour!" he barked.

"Sorry, Mr. Neanderthal, it's been super-busy this morning. How can I help you?"

"I'll tell you how you can help me! You can fix these!" He peeled back his chapped lips to give me a terrifying close-up of his furry, yellow teeth. I cringed.

"I agree – your teeth look pretty awful. Have you been to the dentist?"

"Dentist? Dentist? Don't talk to me about the dentist!" he roared. "He wants to charge me 70 bucks for each tooth he pulls! 70 bucks! Do I look like I'm made of money?!"

"Well, I can't take your teeth out, but what I can do is give you a prescription for some antibiotics and painkillers. That should help settle things down until you get a chance to work something out with your dentist."

"Antibiotics! All you goddamned doctors ever do is prescribe antibiotics! Didn't you hear me? I want these teeth out now!"

"I think you'd better calm down, Mr. Neanderthal. I'm a doctor, not a dentist. How am I supposed to remove your teeth?"

"Don't you know anything? My ex-wife had a cousin with teeth like mine! He got a note from his doctor saying it was an emergency and they took them out for free!"

"Do you know the name of the dental office that did the extractions? Maybe we can give them a call."

"I don't know! Some clinic in the city!"

"I've never heard of that sort of arrangement before, but we can certainly look into it. Did you mention any of this to your dentist?"

"Yeah!"

"What did he say?"

"He said to ask you! How come you don't know about it?"

"I – "

"You're the worst doctor I've ever had! I don't know how you ever got a license! If you don't get my teeth pulled for free right *now*, I'm going to report you to the College of Physicians and Surgeons!"

1, 2, 3, 4, 5, 6, 7, 8, 9, 10 . . . .

"Mr. Neanderthal, I think it's time you found yourself another family doctor."

He jumped off the stretcher and lunged at me. For a second I thought he was going to take a swing.

"Fine! You'll be hearing from the College as well as my lawyer!" He swept by me and stormed out of the department, hurling obscenities over his shoulder. I leaned against the wall and shook my head. *Why on God's green earth do I keep doing this crappy job? I'm clown-hammering myself into oblivion.*

Half an hour later I was wrapping up with another patient when my beeper went off. I dialled switchboard.

"Hi, this is Dr. Gray."

"Hi Dr. Gray," the operator whispered. "Listen, there's a guy out here at the front desk who says he wants to talk to you."

"Just make out a chart and we'll get to him eventually."

"No, he says he's not sick or anything; he just wants to talk to you for a minute."

"This guy wouldn't happen to be Blair Neanderthal, would he?" The last thing I needed was another round of *Sturm und Drang*.

"No, it's not him, thank God."

"Okay, send him in."

In stalked a rough-looking guy in his late 40s. He was wearing a baseball cap, a bomber jacket, black cords and biker boots. His pockmarked face looked vaguely familiar, but I couldn't quite place it. He got right up in my grill and said, "Are you Dr. Gray?"

Is this the part where I get shanked?

"Yes," I replied.

He grabbed my right hand and started pumping it up and down enthusiastically.

"I just wanted to thank you for saving my life two months ago! All the docs down south said I would've been a goner if it hadn't been for you! Thanks!"

Memories flooded back. This fellow had suffered a heart attack and developed a horrendous case of cardiac electrical storm. The doctor on call had paged me *stat* and we worked on him together for several hours. He ended up requiring more than a dozen defibrillations, RSI with post-intubation paralysis and ventilation, thrombolytics, blood thinners, beta-blockers, amiodarone, magnesium, epinephrine, dopamine . . . . He had literally been a one-man Advanced Cardiac Life Support course. It had taken all of our combined knowledge to rescue him. When we finally got him stabilized we had him flown down to a cardiac ICU in southern Ontario via Medevac. And now here he was, alive and well and shaking my hand like there was no tomorrow.

I smiled and patted him on the shoulder.

"You're very welcome, sir," I replied.

And thank you for reminding me why medicine is the best job in the world!

Prima Donna

Quarter to one in the morning. The last outpatient just left the department. My charts are in order. I'm all grokked out. It's time to go home to bed. As I pull on my coat the telephone at switchboard starts ringing. Nine rings later, no one's answered it. That's strange. I go out to investigate and discover there's nobody staffing the switchboard desk. Now that's downright weird – the operator isn't usually more than a few steps away from her phones, and whenever she has to leave the area she always gets someone to cover for her. Maybe she got caught short and had to run to the washroom. Sometimes you're summoned to the throne *most ricky-tick*. The phone is still ringing. What if it's an emergency? I trot over to the desk and pick it up.

"Hello?"

"How busy is the emergency department now?" a nasal female voice demands.

Whoa. Think fast, boyo. You don't want to lie, but on the other hand if you say it's not busy she'll proclaim she's coming in to have her stuffy nose looked at.

"If you have an urgent medical problem or an emergency you'll be seen."

Okay, not that smooth, but acceptable.

"The last time I was there I had to wait 45 minutes before I was finally seen!"

45 minutes? Really? Most other hospitals measure their ER wait times in hours. Were you hoping to beat the rush by showing up at one in the morning?

"I see," I reply blandly, hoping she doesn't recognize my voice.

I guess that response isn't sympathetic enough, because now she's going Medusa on me.

"I want to speak to someone in the emergency department right now!"

Lady, I am the emergency department.

"Hold the line, please," I instruct.

I put her on hold and telephone one of the nurses on the medical floor down the hall.

"If you happen to see the switchboard operator, could you please tell her she has a call on line one? Thanks."

The blinking red light on the console tells me our diva is still on hold. Good. I zip up my coat and leave. I'm grinning like a madman.

Running the Supermarket Gauntlet

"And now, ladies and gentlemen, it's time for another thrilling episode of . . . Supermarket Gauntlet! Watch as our hapless rural physician tries to shop for groceries anonymously! Will he succeed? Of course not! But it's fun to watch him try! Take it away, Dr. Gray!"

Okay, hang on a minute. I don't want to come across as being some sort of Grinchy recluse. Although a number of you may be skeptical (and I'm sure that *last* story didn't help much), please allow me to reassure you that I am not some antisocial curmudgeon freshly sprung from the pages of a Dickens anthology. I honestly do enjoy meeting and greeting people as much as the next guy; it's just that I don't always feel like having a dozen conversations every time I go pick up some eggs. Whenever I want a less communal shopping experience I generally try to go early in the morning – our local supermarket tends to be less congested then. That approach doesn't always work, though. Take today, for example . . . .

Morning inpatient rounds ended 15 minutes earlier than usual, so I decided to do a quick supermarket foray to pick up a few odds and ends. When I arrived I was pleased to see the parking lot was only about one-quarter full. I pulled into a stall and scanned the area. The coast looked clear. I disembarked, ducked my head down low and started speed-walking towards the main entrance. I hadn't gotten more than five paces when a loud voice behind me boomed: "Hey, there's Dr. Gray! Hi Dr. Gray!"

Aargh! Parking lot ambush!

I turned around. It was one of my patients, of course. Like Savoir Faire, they're *everywhere*.

"Hi Mr. Snodgrass."

"Gotta love this weather, eh doc?"

"Absolutely."

"How's your family doing?"

"They're well, thanks. And yours?"

"Great! Say, I'm running low on my little white pills and I was wondering if I could get a refill."

"Your little white pills?"

"Yeah, you know the ones, they're about *this* big . . . ."

"What do you take them for?"

"Geez, that's a good question! I think they're for my cholesterol. No wait, they might be for my blood pressure! Or gout maybe? What colour are gout pills?"

To my credit, I didn't roll my eyes. I hardly ever do that anymore.

"How about you check the name on the bottle when you get home and leave a message for me at my office? Then I'll be able to fax a refill to the drugstore for you."

"Sounds like a plan, doc! You have yourself a great day!"

I bolted inside. As I passed the tiny drugstore near the entrance, Fred the pharmacist waved at me.

"Hi Dr. Gray!"

"Hi Fred, how's it going?"

He motioned me over and dropped his voice to a clandestine whisper.

"Hate to bother you, but would you happen to recall if you told Mr. Johnson you'd phone in a Viagra refill for him yesterday?"

"Oh yes, I did, but then things kind of went sideways on me and I forgot. He can have eight 100 mg tabs with three repeats."

"Thanks!"

"No problem!"

I went to get a shopping cart. One of the women from the hospital auxiliary was sitting at a makeshift desk strategically located right beside the trolley corral.

"Hi Dr. Gray! Care to buy a raffle ticket to support the Disease-of-the-Week Foundation?"

"I'd love to!"

"They're five dollars each."

"I'll take two, please."

I paid my trolley tax, selected one that didn't squeak too much and wheeled it into the store.

Aside from a few nods and waves, my trip down the produce aisle was completely uneventful. Next up was bread. After scoping out some potential candidates, I leaned over and began covertly squeezing loaves. I had a firm grip on a promising loaf of Wonder Bread when I got the distinct feeling someone was watching me. I looked over my shoulder guiltily, expecting to encounter a frowning store clerk.

Fortunately it was just some flaxen-haired, gappy-toothed kid.

"Hey! Dr. Gray! Remember me?"

"Er, no. What's your name again?"

"Ralph! You put a cast on my leg when I broke it last summer."

"Hi, Ralph. How's your leg feeling?"

"Great! I can rollerblade and skateboard and everything now!"

"Awesome."

"So, what are you doing?"

"Shopping."

"How come you're not at work?"

How come you're not at school?

"My office hasn't started yet."

"Oh. What's the matter with that loaf of bread?"

"Nothing."

"So then why were you squeezing it just now?"

"I, uh . . . ."

"Come along, Ralph," his mother called from the far end of the aisle. Leave the peculiar, bread-squeezing doctor alone . . . .

Cereals:

"Hi Dr. Gray!"

"Hi Mrs. MacLeod!"

"Did you get the results of that ultrasound I went for last week?"

"Not yet."

"How about my diabetes test?"

"Um . . . ."

"My cholesterol test?"

"I don't remember."

"My – "

"Usually no news is good news, but if you want you can call my office and they'll look up the results for you."

"Okay, thanks!"

Eggs:

"How's it going, Dr. Gray?"

"Just great, Mr. Polokov. And you?"

"I'm fine. Will your office be open this afternoon? I need to get some travel grants signed."

"We'll be open until about six o'clock."

"I also need some Workers' Compensation forms filled out. How long do you think it'll take you to do them? We're going on a cruise next week and I'd really like to mail them in before we leave."

"If you speak to my receptionist, she'll let you know."

"Thanks!"

Toiletries:

I needed some bathroom supplies, but the recently-jettisoned Blair Neanderthal was parked in the middle of the aisle by the "My First Toothbrush" display. Oh, well, who needs soap, anyway? It's *so* overrated. Detour, detour . . . .

Meat:

"Hey, doc! Thanks for stitching up my finger last week."

"My pleasure."

"It's almost healed already! Do you want to see it?"

"No, that's okay."

"You sure?"

"Positive."

"Actually, would you mind taking a quick peek at it just to make sure it's not getting infected?"

"Okay, let's see . . . . Uh-huh . . . . Looks fine to me."

"Thanks! Say, can you write me a note to give the wife saying I won't be able to do the dishes for the next couple of weeks? Har-har!"

Dairy:

My last stop before checkout was the dairy section. I was reviewing the expiry date on a carton of Lactaid when someone tapped me on the shoulder.

"Dr. Gray, am I ever glad to see you!"

Oh no! The Kiss of Death!

"Hi Mr. Runciter. What's wrong?"

"I've been having one heck of a time with my bladder lately!"

"I see . . . ."

He started pulling up his shirt.
"I think maybe it has to do with my prostate."
"Uh-huh . . . ."
He began fumbling with his belt buckle.
"The last time I got this you ended up having to send me to the urologist."
"Ah . . . ."
He started unbuttoning his pants.
"Mr. Runciter, *what are you doing?!*"
"I figured I'd show you –"
"Not here!"
"Oh, okay doc. Do you want me to drop by your office later?"
"Sure! Five o'clock!"
I skedaddled.

Clearly this incognito *shtick* isn't working out for me. I wonder if it's possible to order my groceries online and have them delivered to my house instead?

Rust Ring

Last Saturday morning one of our local mechanics presented to the ER complaining of a foreign body sensation in his left eye. Apparently on Friday afternoon he had been grinding without safety goggles. Hmm. Never seen *that* before. Our slit lamp was out of commission, so I had him recline on the stretcher in the ophthalmology room and used a magnifying glass to locate the piece of metal embedded in his cornea. I then took one of the single-use topical anaesthetic tubes from the appropriate box in the eye tray and squeezed two drops of tetracaine into the affected eye.

After waiting the customary five or six seconds for the freezing to take effect, I began scraping the surface of his eye with a miniature Alger brush to remove the offending particle. He immediately did a whole-body flinch and bellowed, "Ouch!" I had never seen anyone react like that before. *Geez, what a wimp,* I thought. I added another couple of drops and continued working. This time he sat bolt upright on the stretcher and started rubbing his eye vigorously.

"Ow, doc! I can still feel that!"

"Four drops of tetracaine is more than enough to numb the surface of the eye," I sniffed. Just to be on the safe side, I opened a new tube and put another two or three drops in. "Now please rest your head on the pillow and hold still so I can get this thing out."

Braveheart lay back down reluctantly. After a couple of minutes of scraping I was able to get the metal fragment and its accompanying rust ring off his cornea. It wasn't easy, though – his eye kept watering and he wouldn't stop blinking and squirming around.

Boy, they sure don't make mechanics tough like they used to, I groused to myself when he finally left the department.

At 10:15 on Saturday night I was sitting at the ER desk when the phone rang.

"Hello?"

"Hi doc, it's me, Mike the mechanic."

"Hey, Mike. What's up?"

"I was just wondering how long it'll be before I can see normally again."

"What do you mean?"

"My eye's not as sore as it was before you took that piece of metal out of it, but now everything looks pretty blurry."

"Well, it usually takes a couple of days for the scratch on the surface of the eye to heal."

"Oh, that's good to know. Thanks a million, doc. One last thing – about how long will it be before that black circle in the middle of my eye goes back down to normal size?"

"What?"

"Right now it's way bigger than the one in my right eye. Is that okay?"

"Your pupil is dilated? That doesn't make any sense. Maybe you should come back so I can have another look at you."

Mike returned to the hospital. The ophthalmology room had just been used and needed to be cleaned, so I took a quick look at him out at the ER desk. Sure enough, he had a hugely dilated left pupil. There was no good explanation for it, unless . . . . I went back into the eye room, pulled on a pair of gloves and did the wastepaper basket equivalent of dumpster diving. After a brief search I found the discarded tetracaine tubes I had used on him that morning. Unfortunately, a closer inspection of the labels revealed they weren't tetracaine at all - they were homatropine. Homatropine is used for dilating pupils. It has no topical anaesthetic properties whatsoever. I sifted through the tetracaine box in the cupboard and was only mildly surprised to discover both tetracaine and homatropine tubes in it. True to Murphy's Law, the tubes are almost identical in appearance. My best guess is that the last person to stock the medication cupboard accidentally tossed a handful of homatropine tubes into the tetracaine box. No wonder he'd had such a hard time staying still – he'd been feeling every single scrape and scratch as I worked on the inordinately sensitive surface layer of his eye! The mere thought of it made me want to ralph. I squared my shoulders and went out to face the music.

"Um, Mike, there's something I have to tell you . . . ."

655: Dead, But Dreaming
(Trapped on Jacob's Ladder)

*"As I lay dying, the woman with the dog's eyes
would not close my eyes as I descended into Hades."*

– The spirit of Agamemnon speaking to Odysseus
in Homer's *Odyssey*

*"Is all that we see or seem
but a dream within a dream?"*

– Edgar Allan Poe, *A Dream Within a Dream*

The highways of northern Ontario can extinguish your life in the blink of an eye. One minute you're humming along with the pop star on the radio; the next you're an ugly red smear across a rock cut. Graffiti in flesh and blood. Carrion for the haruspex and obit scavengers. *Did you hear about that horrible accident on 655 last night? What a shame, he was such a nice man . . . .*

Highway 655 is a 60-kilometre strip of desolation that runs between Timmins and the northern branch of the Trans-Canada Highway. Due to chronic staffing shortages, the provincial police have pretty much given up on trying to rigorously enforce the speed limit on it. As a result, 655 has become immensely popular amongst the 18-wheeler crowd. Some days the endless convoys of transports blasting by can make keeping your car out of the ditch a real white-knuckle adventure.

Oddly enough, some nights on 655 you can drive forever and not encounter a single soul. Whenever that happens, my mind has a tendency to wander off and leave my vacant shell steering the car. Although this state bears some resemblance to the automatism that sometimes manifests during minor medical procedures, one key difference is that zombie-driving isn't nearly as closely monitored. As I autopilot down the highway at well over 100 kilometres per hour, a host of half-forgotten memories drift around aimlessly inside my head. Sooner or later my primordial fugue is interrupted by an urgent message from the sector of my neural network tasked with keeping me alive: *Wake up! When's the last time you checked the road?* I usually awaken from my drooling stupor just in time to cringe as a semi passes within a few millimetres of my car. You'd think close calls like that would make me more vigilant, but they don't. Most times I decay back into a torpid, near-REM haze within minutes. It's not that I have a death wish or anything sinister like that – it's just that I'm so tired I can barely keep my eyes open. Sometimes it almost feels as if there are pennies resting on my eyelids.

Strange thoughts seep into my mind at night when I'm in a daze and there's no one else on the highway. Am I really here right now? How can I be certain I didn't fall asleep at the wheel and wrap my car around a tree a few klicks back? Maybe I'm actually pinned under a filigree of twisted metal, coughing up blood and imagining I'm still cruising along a chimeric 655. Could my current existence be nothing more than the terminal hallucinations of a dying brain? Can anoxic neurons spin threads of life out of fear and hope?

Do the dead dream?

Time Flies When You're Having Fun!

Mrs. Charon is in for a routine checkup. I'm running through a review of systems with her.

"Any change in your bowel habits?"
"No."
"Any chest pain?"
"No."
"Shortness of breath?"
"Yes."
"How long have you had that?"
"For a while."
"How long is 'a while'?"
"Oh, a few months, maybe. You did a test on my lungs around the time it started. I had to blow into a machine."
"That was probably a pulmonary function test. When did you do that?"
"Sometime within the past year."

I leaf back through her chart. 2003, 2002, 2001 . . . . Not a pulmonary function test in sight. Nothing. *Nada.*

"Are you sure it was less than a year ago?"
"Yes, doctor."

2000, 1999, 1998 . . . . Zilch. *Bubkes.*

"When did you say you had that test?"
"It was about a month after that time I got really sick and you put that tube down into my lungs and transferred me to Toronto."
"Mrs. Charon, that was over 10 years ago."
"Goodness! Where did the time go?"

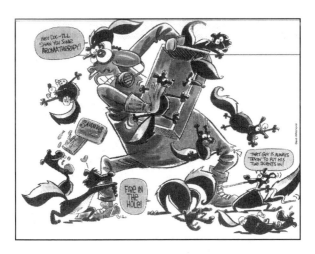

PART THREE
There and Back Again: Return to the Big City

Should I Stay or Should I Go?

Originally when I moved to northern Ontario in 1991 my plan had been to stay for a few years and then hightail it to a warmer latitude. A year later I got married. The following year we started having kids . . . . One amazing decade later Jan and I realized we were approaching a major crossroads in our lives. If we stayed in the north much longer, we'd probably never leave. We had a beautiful home, a great circle of friends and satisfying careers. When she wasn't busy being an elementary school principal Jan took courses, participated in church activities and directed the local community choir. I cycled, snowmobiled, snowboarded, went on canoe trips and wrote. Our daughters were happy with their school lives and extracurricular activities. Why on earth would we ever want to leave? Three words: our extended family. Both sets of parents, as well as Jan's only sister and her family, lived in the Winnipeg area, and we missed them. We wanted our girls to be able to spend more time with their grandparents, aunt, uncle and cousins. We also wanted to be around to assist our parents as they grew older and began meeting new life challenges. In the end, after much soul-searching we decided to pack up the homestead and point our wagons west. But the little town with the polar bears and swans will forever hold a special place in our hearts.

"We Put the K in Kwality!"

July 13, 2004

Dear Kwality Mooovers,

Greetings from Winnipeg. As you know, recently your company moved my family's belongings from northern Ontario to Winnipeg. Although I'm sure Kwality Mooovers usually does stellar work, unfortunately this particular move did not go so smoothly. The following is a list of some of the problems we encountered:

- I suspect your employee Billy-Bob *("Moooving Consultant")* didn't take his Ritalin the day he came to survey the contents of our house, because he certainly didn't appear to be paying attention to anything. Nevertheless, his quote of $7,738.01 was better than your competitor's so we awarded the contract to your company.
- Rather than being packed on June 28 and moved on June 29 as I had stipulated when I booked the move, we were erroneously scheduled to be packed on June 29 and moved on June 30 instead.
- The "packing crew" sent to our house on June 29 consisted of one 67-year-old woman who had been sweet-talked out of retirement. She had been given instructions to pack all of our breakables in the morning and then drive to a home in another community to do their packing in the afternoon. She took one look at the number of items in our house and immediately telephoned to cancel her afternoon assignment. Despite putting in a solid day's work she was unable to finish the job because it was simply far too much for one person. My wife and I had to work well into the night in order to complete the packing.
- On June 30 the moving team arrived more than two hours late with a semi-trailer that was already half-filled with someone else's furniture. It therefore came as no surprise later in the day when they ran out of space in the trailer for our belongings. As your company was unable to procure any other vehicles that day, they had to cram the overflow into our garage. While they were busy doing that, one of the movers (a jolly fellow with no shirt who spent much of the day drinking beer) broke our most expensive lamp. Several other items got badly scratched, dinged, and stained during the transfer process. After the crew finally departed, a subsequent tour of our home revealed a host of overlooked articles. My wife and I had to move these items to the garage ourselves.
- Although we had been promised the movers would be finished by 1:00 p.m. at the latest, they in fact did not leave until after 9:30 p.m. This forced us to alter our travel plans and forfeit the hotel reservations we had made for Thunder Bay. We also had to ask the new owner of our home to postpone his possession date, which was a nuisance for him.

- Due to the various delays our July 1 Canada Day plans with family and friends in Winnipeg were ruined.
- Shortly after our arrival in Winnipeg I was notified that Billy-Bob had underestimated the weight of the shipment by approximately *4,000 pounds* and we would have to pay $11,841.44 on delivery instead of the $7,738.01 originally quoted. This represented an astounding *53 percent markup!* I immediately contacted your head office about this mind-boggling discrepancy and was told the only way the driver would release our furniture would be if we paid him the previously agreed upon amount plus an additional 10 percent. I was also advised your company's CEO and I would have to "work out the difference." When I called your chief executive about the matter he said (and I quote) "Don't worry about it – we just want you to be happy!" *Bobby McFerrin much?*
- Instead of arriving on July 3 at 9:00 a.m., the moving truck didn't show up until July 4 at noon. This was highly inconvenient because my wife had to leave Winnipeg on the morning of the 4th to attend a course, so she was not able to be present for the initial unloading and unpacking.
- Only two people were sent to do the unpacking. One was an elderly man and the other was a teenager. They worked from noon until 1:00 a.m., and it would have taken them an additional four or five hours had I not been carting boxes and hauling furniture right alongside them. I even had to assist in carrying our grand piano up the front steps because the young apprentice would almost certainly have been crippled for life had he been forced to continue lifting his end of it all by himself.
- More than 40 boxes had not been tagged by the team in Ontario, so the check-off process was grossly inaccurate. In addition to that, a number of articles that arrived safely (e.g., our washer, dryer, fridge, stove) were not even recorded on any of the inventory lists as having been sent. Had they not arrived, I would undoubtedly have had a difficult time getting them replaced because your Claims Department labours under the delusion that if an item is not listed on the manifest then it doesn't exist.
- Although it was supposed to be a "complete unpack," when the unpacking "crew" left there were still more than 30 unopened

boxes scattered throughout the house. They said they'd return within a couple of days to dispose of the empty boxes and advise me of the final weight (no one seemed to have a hot clue as to the actual weight of our load), but I've seen neither hide nor hair of them since.
- I am now in receipt of an invoice from your company soliciting the balance of the $11,841.44 you claim I owe you. With all due respect, I don't think so. Have a nice day.

Sincerely,

Donovan Gray *("Moooving Victim")*

Where's Waldo?

"It is astonishing just how much of what we are can be tied to the beds we wake up in in the morning, and it is astonishing how fragile that can be."
– Excerpt from *Coraline*, by Neil Gaiman

Last year our family moved from northern Ontario to Winnipeg, where I've been working part-time in an emergency department as well as in an Urgent Care centre. I return to Ontario one week per month to do clinic and ER locum tenens work. This means I currently have three jobs in two provinces. My shifts in Winnipeg are a screwball mixture of days, evenings and nights. Most are eight hours long, but some are 10. In Ontario my stretches of ER call are anywhere from 24 to 72 hours in duration.

Human beings are not well-equipped to work irregular hours for prolonged intervals. This is in part because shift work wreaks havoc on our natural circadian rhythm. As a result, over time the perpetual flitting between the various shift categories exacts a heavy physiological toll. Diet, sleep, fitness levels and even relationships often develop significant fault lines as the tectonic plates of our professional and private lives crush against one another. For those of us who practice the art of mending broken bodies, night shifts are universally acknowledged to be the most difficult to adapt to. I can handle two or three consecutive graveyards without incurring too much additional stress, but anything more than that starts to make me feel like I'm about to join the ranks of the undead. Whenever I finally revert to regular daytime hours after a long stretch of nights I always half-expect to burst into flames the moment sunlight makes contact with my skin. Perhaps I've read *'Salem's Lot* one time too many . . . .

On a more scientific note, I recently came across a study that suggested shift workers suffer higher rates of accidents, heart attacks, strokes and depression than people who work more conventional hours. Based on what I've seen over the years, I'd say there's probably a lot of truth to that theory.

Where I sleep prior to starting a shift depends on my schedule. If I'm working days then I'll sleep my nights in our bedroom upstairs. If I'm scheduled to work nights I prefer to siesta in the basement because it's usually quieter down there. If the kids are raising Cain and preventing me from banking a few hours of sleep before my night shift, sometimes I'll drive over to my parents' house for some shut-eye. When I'm working in Ontario I stay in the locum house or apartment if either one is available, but if they're already occupied then I bivouac in one of the local motels. Lastly, all three hospitals have designated quiet rooms that can be used for late-night catnaps when things settle down. If my count is correct, that's nine different pillows my head makes contact with on a fairly regular basis.

Sometimes I'm gently shaken awake by Jan or one of my daughters. More commonly, I'm resurrected by the wakeup chirp of my Pocket PC or the buzz of an alarm clock. In Ontario the nurses usually telephone when they need me to come to the ER at night, but occasionally they get in touch with me via my pager. If I'm dozing in one of the hospital nap rooms my *réveillé* tends to be a knock on the door.

Once in a while I'll wake with a start in a darkened room and have no idea where I am. Am I at home? My parents' house? The locum apartment? A motel? One of the hospitals? Which one? As I fumble to get my bearings, a second tsunami of questions hits. Am I on call? What time is it? Did I sleep through an alarm? Am I late for something?

What the hell is going on? It's hard to describe the feeling of complete disorientation. I suspect it's analogous to what a golem experiences the moment it becomes sentient. Shift work. Not for the faint of heart!

Gyne Stretcher at Midnight

G1
P0
20 weeks
Cramping
Bleeding
Passing a large clot
Not a clot
A fetus
Dead
Not dead
Stirring
Pink Cronenberg mass
Legs now kicking
Thin arms reaching
Instinctively trying to return
Reenter the womb
Sanctuary
False hope
No hope
Dying
Slowly
Mouth opening
Silent scream
I stare
Frozen
Helpless
Powerless
The horror
The horror . . . .

Lost Soul

Arun was my organic chemistry lab partner back in pre-med. I didn't mind the organic chem course work, but I sure hated the labs. As far as I was concerned, pouring foul-smelling hydrocarbons from one beaker into another for three hours every Monday morning was sheer torture. During the first month students worked solo, but after that we were partnered up. Fortunately for me, I got to work with Arun.

Which adjectives best describe Arun? Intelligent and well-organized would probably be first out of the gate, followed closely by soft-spoken, generous and athletic. He had a dry sense of humour and an impish grin. One thing's for sure – he was the best lab partner a slacker like me could ever have hoped for. I'd usually show up five minutes late, flop down beside him at our work station and ask what was going on. He'd take a break from pipetting the methyl-ethyl-whatever and patiently describe the experiment I was supposed to have read up on over the weekend.

"Cool," I'd reply. "So, what do you need me to do?" I'm pretty sure the only thing he ever needed me to do was stay out of his way, but he always managed to come up with some little job to keep me busy so the instructor wouldn't realize what a useless twit I was.

In the fall of 1983 Arun and I were both accepted into the Faculty of Medicine at the University of Manitoba in Winnipeg. I didn't see much of him during the first two years of the program, but on those occasions when our paths did cross he seemed fine. Halfway through our third year we were all promoted to the rank of "baby clerk" and dumped on the wards. The sudden increase in pressure proved too much for some, and a handful of my classmates imploded.

Arun was one of the first casualties. There was no warning - one day he was with us and the next he was gone. Rumour had it he had been diagnosed with schizophrenia. Back then my friends and I thought schizophrenia was just an exotic word that lived in psychiatry textbooks, not something that could actually reach into our world and touch us. It didn't seem possible. We should have sought him out and offered moral support, but most of us were too busy trying to stay afloat ourselves to worry about a fallen comrade. The general philosophy of most medical schools in the 1980s could probably be summarized in three words: Sink or swim. As Arun sank, the rest of us continued dog-paddling ferociously. No one looked back.

Over the years there were sporadic Arun sightings. Once a classmate had a meal at a restaurant and Arun waited on his table. Occasionally someone would bump into him at a movie theatre or in a grocery store. Having a meaningful conversation with him became increasingly difficult as his thought patterns grew more tangential. Each encounter left one with the distinct impression that he was slowly disintegrating. It was as though tiny fragments of his personality were breaking off and floating away. Eventually Arun became withdrawn and dishevelled-looking. *Poor Arun*, we'd say, as we hurried to our next clinic. *We should go visit him.* Then one of us would get paged and we'd race away to deal with the crisis.

A year after completing my training I moved to northern Ontario. Things got even busier for me. I started a practice, got married, became a father . . . . Life was good. I forgot all about my former lab partner.

Last summer we moved back to Winnipeg. Over the Christmas holidays we were invited to a friend's house for a Boxing Day brunch. Seven of my former classmates were there. While our children chased each other around the house we gathered in the kitchen and reminisced about our years in medical school. All of a sudden I remembered Arun.

"Hey," I said, turning to our host, "when's the last time you saw Arun?"

His smile froze.

"Didn't you hear?" he asked. "Arun left home depressed one day last March and never came back. They pulled his body out of the Red River six weeks later. He drowned."

I'm sorry I wasn't there for you, Arun.

In memory of Arun Sud *(1963–2004)*

Arun's family would like to hear from any of his classmates or others who knew him while he was a student. His family can be reached by e-mail at gitasudca@yahoo.ca.

A scholarship fund has been set up in Arun's memory through the Manitoba Schizophrenia Society. The scholarship will be awarded to a student with a mental illness pursuing university or college. Anyone wishing to make a donation can contact the Manitoba Schizophrenia Society at (204) 786-1616, email info@mss.mb.ca, or regular mail: 100 - 4 Fort Street, Winnipeg, MB, R3C 1C4.

The Cost of Letting Go

In the opening pages of *The Bad Beginning* (the first book of Lemony Snicket's *A Series of Unfortunate Events*), the Baudelaire children are roaming along a beach. Violet is holding a stone in her hand. She spots a figure in the distance hurrying towards them, and in an instant she intuitively knows he is the bearer of terrible news. Eventually he arrives and informs them that their parents have just perished in a fire.

As the numb Baudelaire orphans get ready to follow the emissary back down the beach and into the unknown, Violet realizes she is still holding the stone. When she first picked it up, her life was idyllic. Now it is utterly alien. The stone was present when *before* became *after*. It links her new self to her former self. She lets it fall to the ground.

As parents, we have a natural tendency to want to keep our children nestled under our protective wings forever. We are, of course, aware that this is neither possible nor desirable, but part of us is still tempted to do it anyway.

My children are now starting to take their first unaccompanied steps out into the world. In the past, Jan and I have always been there in one way or another – if not front and centre, then at least as a shadowy presence on the periphery, carefully monitoring them and ensuring every situation met our stringent safety standards.

Now, as we stand on the verge of a brave new world of Facebook, sleepovers, preteen dances and "you can drop me off here, Dad, you don't have to come inside," we must struggle to strike a new balance. Too much liberty isn't good, but neither is not enough.

Whenever my girls are off somewhere that isn't 100 percent guaranteed safe and sound, I get a little nervous. If they're five minutes late getting back from riding their bikes to the corner store, my paranoia runs amok. There's been an accident, they got lost, some psycho killer nabbed them, whatever. I start identifying with Violet Baudelaire:

Is this the moment when my *before* becomes *after*?

Then I give my head a good shake and I'm okay. And two minutes later they're home, laughing and telling me about the cool bird's nest they found.

They're going to be just fine. I'm the one who may have a few rough years coming up.

Doctor Lockout

Last Thursday I worked an ER shift that ended at 1:00 a.m. As is often the case, the department went ballistic during the final hour and I ended up staying late to help tie up loose ends. My home is at the opposite end of the city, so by the time I finally pulled into our garage it was after 2:00.

As I gathered up my junk and made my way to the inner garage door I did a quick sleep calculation. My next shift started at 8:00 a.m., which meant that if I went to bed right away I'd get about four hours of shut-eye. Not ideal, but certainly not Armageddon.

I gripped the doorknob and twisted. It didn't budge. What the heck? We never lock the inner garage door. I tried again. Nothing. I checked my keys. None for that door. To make matters worse, I didn't have my front door key because I'd loaned it to one of my daughters earlier in the week. I tried knocking loudly.

"Hello? Jan? Girls?" No reply. That was no surprise – my wife and kids sleep so soundly, you'd think they'd been anaesthetized. "Let me in!" I yowled. No response. Honking the horn and ringing the doorbell didn't work either. I sat on the steps, temporarily stymied. Then I got a brainwave – telephone them! I was pawing through my briefcase for my cell phone when I remembered I'd left it in its charging unit in the kitchen. Rats! There was only one solution. I hopped in my truck and drove off in search of a phone.

I thought I'd find one right away, but 10 minutes later there was still no phone booth in sight. I continued driving. Soon the big blue hospital sign of Brigadoon General appeared on the horizon. I don't work there, but I figured they'd probably have a couple of pay phones in the lobby of their ER. I coasted into a parking spot and jogged inside.

Much like our own waiting room, theirs had the industry-standard 30 or more people thumbing through magazines older than the Dead Sea Scrolls, glancing at their watches and shooting the occasional dirty look at the triage nurse. She didn't seem to be the least bit perturbed by the negative vibes being slung in her direction, though. To tell you the truth, she looked like one tough cookie. I approached her Plexiglas-fortified bunker and cleared my throat.

"Excuse me," I began.

"Yes?"

"Could I please get some change to use your pay phone?"

"Does this look like a 7-11 to you?"

"Er . . . ."

"No change!" She then jumped up and pointed at some poor slob in the waiting room who was drunkenly trying to light a cigarette. "Hey, you! Can't you read? No smoking in here!"

The last thing I wanted was to be in her way when she leaped over her desk and body-slammed the guy, so I did a quick U-turn and beetled over to the area with the telephones.

It turned out the phones accepted plastic. I put my card in and dialled our number.

Ring . . . .

Ring . . . .

Ring . . . .

"Hi, this is the Gray residence. We're not home right now, so please leave a message at the sound of the beep."

"Jan, it's me. You've locked me out! It's 2:30 in the morning! Wake up and let me in!" No response. I hung up and tried again.

Ring . . . .

Ring . . . .

Ring . . . .

"Hi, this is the Gray residence. We're not home right now . . . ."
I could feel my jaw begin to clench. I took one of those deep Zen-Master-seeks-inner-peace breaths and dialled Jan's cell.

Ring . . . .
Ring . . . .
Ring . . . .

"Your call has been forwarded to a voicemail service that has not been activated by the customer. Please try again later."

"Aargh!!"

Attila the Nurse skewered me with a glare.

"Keep it quiet over there!"

Six or seven tries later I gave up and drove home. It was now 3:00. I sat in my truck and contemplated my options:

1. Go to my parents' place, wake them up and stay there until the morning.
2. Rent a motel room.
3. Sleep in the truck.

Then inspiration struck. I decided to get our ladder, climb to the second storey and pound on our bedroom window until Jan woke up. Gee, why didn't I think of that before? Maybe because the idea was completely insane. In any case, a few minutes later I was in our pitch-black backyard leaning a 20-foot ladder against the wall and hoping the police weren't planning to patrol our neighbourhood anytime soon.

I was halfway up the ladder when a thought occurred to me: *I wonder if Jan remembered to lock the patio door before she went to bed?* My wife tends to be a little security-challenged sometimes. I descended, walked over to the glass door and pulled. It slid open with a sigh.

Later that morning when we got up Jan commented that I had been grinding my teeth in my sleep again.

I Sure Do Love Ol' What's Her Name!

Twice a week I head down to the local YMCA in a desperate attempt to build up my puny muscles. So far it's not working. I'm not much of a social butterfly, so I don't usually have too many conversations while I'm there. I do enjoy people-watching, though. From what I've seen, the Y is populated by four main phenotypes:

1. The Alphas
Fit, tanned and orthodontically perfect; they always look as though they just blew in from a tropical photo shoot for the next issue of *Vogue* or *GQ*. Alphas socialize almost exclusively with other alphas. I often wonder where they go when they leave the gym. Back to Mount Olympus, probably.

2. The Muscle Heads
Easy to spot. Just look for the pumped-up gorillas making grunty noises as they bench press stacks of weights heavier than your average minivan.

3. The I'm-Here-Because-My-Doctor-Prescribed-Regular-Exercise Gang
This group is distinguished by their silver hair and Olivia Newton John-style headbands. Hey folks, what's up with the cheesy 1975 fashion accessory? Not even the steroid-gargling Conans sweat enough to require headbands!

4. The Average Joes
Middle-aged *schlubs* like yours truly half-heartedly fighting the Battle of the Bulge. Most of us are getting our butts kicked.

A couple of months ago I attended a story-reading event put on by Ellen's grade six class. It was held in the McNally Robinson bookstore café. Each student sat at a table with members of their family and awaited their turn to go to the podium and read a story they had written. Near the end of the evening I spotted a familiar face in the crowd. At first I couldn't quite place him, but a few minutes later I realized he was one of the Schwarzeneggers from the gym (see category 2 above). He was sitting with one of Ellen's classmates. Based on their respective ages, I concluded that he was probably her father. Ellen mentioned the girl's name was Nicole. I filed the random bit of information away under

Miscellaneous and turned my attention back to my family.

The following week I was at the gym flailing away at some god-awful pectoralis-strengthening contraption when the fellow I had noticed at the bookstore sat down on the machine opposite me.

"Hey," I said, "Do you have a relative in grade six at École Française?" He looked at me blankly. Undaunted, I pressed on. "I was at the story-reading at McNally Robinson with my daughter last Friday and I thought I saw you there with one of her classmates." He continued staring at me like I had two heads. I swear, he wasn't even blinking. That must hurt your eyes after a while. Eventually I shrugged my shoulders. "Sorry, my mistake. It's just that I was almost positive I saw you sitting with a girl with wavy red hair near the front of the café. My daughter told me her name, but I can't remember it now. I think it started with N."

The vegetative look persisted. Clearly our "conversation" was on life support. It was time to pull the plug.

"Must have been a doppelgänger," I concluded. I was about to move on to the next machine when his eyes suddenly registered a glimmer of recognition. A split second later they widened excitedly and his mouth formed the universal 'O' of surprised discovery. It's a miracle Archimedes didn't appear in a puff of smoke and yell *"Eureka!"*

"Oh, you must mean *Nicole!* Yeah, yeah, we were there! That was us, all right! Yeah!"

"So, how are you two related?"

"She's my daughter."

Is There a Doctor on Board?

I fly fairly often. As a result, I've heard the dreaded refrain *"If there's a doctor on board, please identify yourself to a member of the cabin crew"* more times than I care to remember. The last time it happened I was wedged into a window seat. By the time the pleasant but glacier-slow elderly couple sitting beside me managed to extricate themselves from their seats and let me pass, several people had already beaten me to the scene. A woman in her early 20s was slumped in the aisle near the back of the plane. She appeared to be unconscious. In addition to the usual rubberneckers and gawkers, she was surrounded by a trio of flight attendants and a distinguished-looking gentleman in horn-rimmed glasses. As I threaded my way through the rabble I reflexively began working on a list of potential diagnoses and their respective treatments. There were several things I would need to determine as quickly as possible. Was she breathing adequately? Did she have a pulse? If so, was it regular? What was her blood pressure? Could she have had an arrhythmia? A seizure? Ruptured ectopic? Diabetic coma? Chances were it was just a simple faint, but even if it was, did she injure herself when she fell? It all started with a set of vital signs, but there was just one problem – I couldn't get past the flight attendants and the Peter O'Toole lookalike. He seemed to be holding court.

"To the trained eye, this is quite obviously a textbook case of vasovagal syncope," he pontificated, "which of course is the proper medical term for the phenomenon you will almost certainly recognize by its far more colloquial name – a fainting spell." He beamed. His audience was enthralled by the impromptu lecture. No one seemed to be examining the woman on the floor, though.

"Excuse me, I'm an ER doctor," I offered.

"Not to worry, my young colleague; everything's under control. I'm a doctor, too," he responded. He turned back to the attendants. "Vasovagal syncope is usually the result of – "

"Sorry to interrupt," I interrupted, "but is she breathing okay?"

"Breathing?" he said. "Breathing? Um . . . ." He bent down and shook her arm. A few seconds later she stirred and let out a groan. "Yes, of course! She's breathing superbly!"

"Oh, that's a relief," I replied. "What's her pulse?"

"Pulse? Er . . . ." He began fidgeting with his tie. I was just about to step past him when the woman opened her eyes and sat up.

"I think I just fainted," she announced. "I do that every now and then."

Our patient was fine. It was time for me to return to my seat. Before I left, though, I was dying to know something. I turned to the other physician.

"Just out of curiosity, what type of medicine do you practice?"
"Psychiatry."

Fit for Duty

A couple of weeks ago I did another rural locum in northern Ontario. My first patient of the day at the No Family Doctor Clinic was a scruffy-looking fellow in his late 20s.

"Hi Mr. Capgras, I'm Dr. Gray. How can I help you today?"
"I need you to sign this form saying I'm healthy."
"Who is it for?"
"The military. I'm applying to get in and they want confirmation I'm fit for duty."
"Are you healthy?"
"Yep. You just need to put your initials here and here and sign at the bottom." He very helpfully offered me a pen. My Spidey senses started tingling. I deposited the pen on the desk and scanned through the form. They did indeed want verification he was in good physical and psychological condition. Unfortunately, that's pretty hard to do when you've only known someone for half a minute. He seemed to be in reasonable physical shape, but did he have all his marbles? I recalled an old pearl of wisdom from medical school: *When in doubt, ask the patient.*

"Perhaps I should be more specific. Do you have any physical health problems?"
"Nope."
"What about mental health problems?"
"Not really . . . ."
"How about in the past?"
"Um . . . ."

Pearl of wisdom from 15 years of clinical practice: *When all else fails, check the chart.*

"Do you mind if I quickly review your file?"
"Er . . . ."

I opened it and started leafing through. It didn't take long to spot certain glaring trends.

"Gee, it says here you've had long-standing issues with panic attacks, substance abuse, alcoholism, obsessive-compulsive disorder and multiple personality disorder."

"Really?"

"It also mentions at least five different admissions to psychiatric hospitals within the past two years."

"No way."

"Way."

"I forgot."

"According to the most recent discharge summary, you just got out last week."

"Oh."

A slightly awkward silence settled over the room. Finally, my patient cleared his throat and spoke.

"Does this mean you won't be able to sign my form?"

Ode to a Carrot Juice Enema

I'm sure there must be some good naturopaths out there, but I've yet to run into one. How's *that* for an opening salvo?

Every month a gastroenterologist from a nearby city has an endoscopy clinic at one of the rural hospitals I work at. For colonoscopy the bowels need to be as empty as possible in order to permit a good evaluation of the mucosa. To that end, patients are asked to take two oral Fleet phosphosoda laxatives on the evening prior to their procedure. The Fleets are remarkably effective at evacuating the bowels and cost only $6.99 each.

Recently a naturopath in the area began offering carrot juice enemas as an alternative to the traditional bowel prep. Carrot juice enemas cost $120. As if that wasn't bad enough, the damn things don't work. Instead of inducing the usual 10 or more bowel movements, the carrot juice regimen produces a paltry one or two. One or two BMs aren't nearly enough to clean out the average person's colon. Shortly after this new "service" became available, patients started showing up for their colonoscopies with their bowels full of carrot juice and crap. The gastroenterologist would only be able to advance the scope about six inches before running into a solid wall of orange sludge. The procedure would then have to be aborted and rescheduled for a later date. We'd ask people who'd had previous scopes how in the world they figured one or two poops could possibly clear them out when the standard regimen had made them go at least 10 times. *"Well, to tell you the truth doc, I was kind of wondering how that was going to work myself...."* Eventually our exasperated consultant began giving his patients free colonoscopic snapshots of the gooey, carroty conglomerate in their bowels so they'd at least have some hard evidence should they attempt to obtain a refund. *Madre de Dios!* Like the saying goes, a fool and his money are soon parted.

Speaking of fools and their money, another naturopath some of my patients liked to frequent claimed to be able to assess their bio-spiritual *chi* by closing her eyes and doing this weird hand-fluttering thing around their bodies. After a couple of minutes of humming and swaying she'd come out of her little trance and proclaim that they were dangerously low in xenon or antimatter or whatever. And you thought psychic mass spectrometry didn't exist! Silly you! A vanishingly small bottle of the life-saving element or mineral their soul so desperately craved would always be available for a mere $75. Cheap like borscht! Oddly enough, the bottles all looked the same to me. I saw a lot of them because after leaving their mystic consultations my patients would invariably rush straight to my office requesting laboratory confirmation of their new diagnosis. *"Do I really have a titanium deficiency, doc? Is that bad?"* I was often tempted to have the mysterious fluid in the bottles analyzed to see what it really was. Probably carrot juice. A real bar-goon, folks. *Ka-ching!*

Oh Lordy, here comes the hate mail!

When Your Compassion Runs Out

I was in a toxic mood. Why? Because I'd worked 12 of the last 14 days. Because it was my third graveyard in a row and I was beat.

Because the shift had been snakebit from the get-go and I was tired of dealing with crackheads, criminals, and bacchants. Sometimes prolonged immersion in the seamy underbelly of a city can be a little soul-destroying. Do it for too long and you start to grow steel behind your eyes. Cripes, who cares what the reasons were? The bottom line is I was fresh out of compassion.

I picked up the next patient's chart. The triage note indicated she was a 35-year-old shoplifting suspect who had been involved in an altercation with some security guards. *Great*, I thought, *just what I need. A maenad*. I knocked on the door and entered the treatment room.

The tall, thin woman curled up on the stretcher had spiky black hair and pinched features. She was sporting an angry purple bruise on her right cheek.

"Are you the doctor?"

"Yes."

"About time." She uncoiled her body and pointed at her cheek. "I want this documented. These too." She rolled up her sleeves to reveal several abrasions on her wrists and forearms.

"What happened?" I asked.

"Some guys jumped me."

"When did this occur?"

"About six hours ago."

"Where?"

"Is this really necessary?" she hissed. "I already played 20 Questions with the cops as well as that nosy bitch at the front desk. I don't feel like doing the same thing with you, too."

Hoo-boy, was that ever the wrong answer. Now we were going to do this the hard way.

"As a matter of fact, it is necessary," I replied coldly. "I need to review all the details myself to ensure nothing gets missed. If that doesn't suit you, you're welcome to get your medical care somewhere else."

She shot me a poisonous look, then grumbled, "It happened at the Cost-Savers store downtown."

"Why did these people attack you?"

"How should I know?"

It was obvious she didn't want to admit she had been caught shoplifting. I should have just cut her some slack and dropped the subject, but for some reason I was bound and determined to extract a confession. I continued baiting her.

"So a mob of complete strangers tackled you in the middle of a busy department store for no particular reason?"

"They were security guards."

"What made them pick you?"

"I guess they must have thought I was shoplifting or something."

"Were you?"

Checkmate. Mongoose victorious.

She hung her head and stared at the floor for a few seconds. When she looked up again, her eyes were glazed with tears.

"Yeah, I was," she whispered. "I tried to steal a cheap watch. But why'd they have to hurt me so bad? It's not like I was going to fight them for it. I only took it because I was broke and hungry and I didn't know what else to do . . . ."

It was one of the lowest moments of my medical career.

Guilt

"The only thing that burns in hell is the part of you that won't let go of your life."

– Louis' interpretation of a Meister Eckhart concept in *Jacob's Ladder*

When I woke up in the ER on-call nap room at 6:00 this morning Mr. Trapper was sitting at my bedside. I always flinch when that happens.

"You're not really here," I said. "You're dead."

"Well, you don't have to be so rude about it," he grumbled.

"I'm sorry," I apologized. "It's just that sometimes I get tired of reminding you."

His shoulders slumped, which made me feel guilty. I tried to rationalize: *Don't be ridiculous. The dead have no feelings.*

"Why do you keep coming back?" I asked.

He pulled a handkerchief out of his translucent pocket and wiped his forehead.

"You know why."

"Why?"

"I want to live."

"I'm sorry Mr. Trapper, but much as I'd like to, I can't change what happened."

He blew his nose and put the handkerchief away.

"It wasn't any fun dying alone on the bathroom floor, doc. They didn't find me for a week. I *trusted* you. This whole thing is so unfair," he said quietly.

I looked directly into his hollow eyes.

"I truly am sorry," I said.

I stepped over his shimmering suitcase, entered the hallway and gently pulled the door closed behind me.

"It's so unfair," he whispered as it clicked shut.

Time to Go

Recently a pleasant 95-year-old widow named Rose presented to our ER after a brief episode of chest pressure. The discomfort subsided en route to the hospital and never recurred. One of my colleagues examined her and ordered a battery of tests, all of which turned out to be normal. Later that evening he reviewed the results with the patient and her son and recommended she stay in our department overnight for cardiac monitoring. Rose was not interested in any form of aggressive resuscitation, but she didn't mind a brief period of observation. After helping her get settled in for the night, Rose's son departed saying he'd be back at nine in the morning to take his mother home.

At 4:00 a.m. Rose awoke from a deep sleep and rang the call bell. When her nurse arrived Rose said, "Laura, it's time for me to go."

Laura glanced at her watch in the half-light and replied, "Oh, it's not time yet, ma'am; it's only four o'clock. Your son said he'd come get you around nine."

Rose gazed up at her nurse through sibylline eyes. She clasped

Laura's hands in hers and patted them gently.

"You don't understand, dear. It's time for me to *go*." She then smiled, folded her arms across her chest and closed her eyes. On the cardiac monitor above the head of the bed Rose's heart rate plummeted from 80 to 50 to 20 to flatline in less than a minute. And just like that she was gone, with a cryptic little Mona Lisa smile still fixed on her lips.

Piece of Cake

Joanna is a seasoned Winnipeg emergency room RN. We're talking old-school here. Hard-boiled. Always prepared. The original Swiss Army nurse. Recently she worked a long string of 12-hour nights. On Saturday morning when she got home she was exhausted. She knew she needed to get some sleep because she was scheduled to host her twin daughters' 8th birthday party that afternoon and her husband was out of town. Unfortunately, between household chores and all the pre-party preparations she never made it to bed. At 2:00 p.m. the guests arrived. The kids had a great time running around and playing games. At 4:30 they sang *Happy Birthday*, cut the cake and opened gifts. By then Joanna was wishing she had a pair of toothpicks to help prop her eyelids open. She had only enough energy left to smile blearily at anyone who approached and croak, "Would you like some cake?"

At 5:15 the last guest left. Our sleep-deprived heroine tidied the house, made supper, helped her kids pack overnight bags and dropped them off at their grandmother's. She then got herself ready and drove to the hospital for the last of her 7:30 p.m. to 7:30 a.m. night shifts.

By midnight she was a complete zombie. To make matters worse, the elderly gentleman she was trying to triage was a rambler.

"How can we help you tonight, sir?"

"Well ma'am, in the summer of '52 I injured my back while I was working in the oil patch out in Alberta, but in those days there wasn't no such thing as Compensation so I just kept plugging away until one morning the damned thing just seized up on me and I couldn't even get out of bed so I had to get my best friend Wilbur Mercer to drive me to the nearest hospital and the doc there took one look at me all bent over like a pretzel and he said . . ."

Joanna's eyelids began to droop.

". . . my back was just plain old worn out and there wasn't really a whole heck of a lot he could do for me except for maybe some kind of steroid injection thing but he sent me off to see a sawbones anyway and believe it or not that doc operated on me the very next day and lucky for me he did because . . ."

Joanna's eyes drifted shut. As she quietly snoozed while sitting upright in her chair at the triage desk, the Midnight Rambler carried on with his ever-so-precise and focused history.

". . . within a month or so I was back at work on them rigs like nothing had ever happened and that's how I ended up with this here little scar right above my tailbone. Once in a while when there's a change in the weather it aches something fierce for a few hours and I have to take a couple of them Tylenols to settle it down. Tonight I got to thinking about it and I started wondering if there might be a good medical explanation for why that happens. But that's not actually the real reason why I'm here tonight. No, ma'am, the main reason I decided I should come see a doctor tonight is because about 40 years ago I was on top of my neighbour Phil Resch's barn helping him patch a hole that had been leaking for pretty near a month and best I can figure I must have slipped on some pigeon poop because wouldn't you know it all of a sudden I took a spill right off that goldarn roof and . . . Ma'am?" Our patient had just realized his nurse was asleep. He gently nudged her arm. "Ma'am, are you okay?"

Joanna lurched awake, bug-eyed and completely disoriented.

"WOULD YOU LIKE SOME CAKE?"

Skunked

One morning this spring Jan glanced up from her newspaper to see a skunk ambling across our backyard. We're accustomed to seeing all sorts of wildlife in our neighbourhood, but we had never witnessed a skunk before. She grabbed my camera and snapped a picture of it. That evening my daughters and I viewed the image and marvelled. It's not every day you see a skunk, even if it's just on the LCD screen of a digital Canon.

The next morning the skunk reappeared at exactly the same time. We all stared as she casually meandered around for several minutes before disappearing into our neighbour's backyard through a crack in the fence.

"I think we should do something about this," Jan announced.

"Nah," I responded. "She's probably just passing through."

The skunk was back at seven o'clock the following morning. And the next. And the next . . . . She was so regular you could set your watch by her. My daughters took to calling her Skunky. Not long after that the words *pet skunk* began creeping into their conversations.

"We definitely need to do something about this," Jan would mutter darkly.

"Maybe she lives at the neighbour's place," I'd reply, fingers crossed.

One morning Skunky didn't show up at her appointed time. She missed her cameo the following day, too. Two months passed with no further skunk sightings.

"Told you," I'd say smugly from time to time. "She was just passing through."

Jan would just roll her eyes.

Two weeks ago Jan and I were looking through the living room window at a peculiar strip of shredded grass in our front yard when, lo and behold, Skunky sashayed into view.

"I wonder where she's been?" I pondered aloud.

Jan banged on the window. Skunky jumped in alarm and zipped down a hitherto-unnoticed hole in the earth where our garden meets the concrete of our front steps. *Uh-oh*. Jan turned to me with one eyebrow raised. That's always a bad sign.

"Just passing through, eh?"

"I'll call pest control in the morning."

The pest control company said they'd be out to set a trap in a few days.

The following evening I was updating a family photo album in our living room when Skunky emerged from her den. For several minutes I watched her scratch great big holes in our lawn in search of whatever it is skunks call supper. Eventually I got bored and returned to my picture sorting. The next time I glanced up there were eight baby skunks cavorting on the grass in front of our garden. I nearly choked. The miniature black-and-white furballs were having a rollicking good time chasing one another's tails, pouncing like kittens and rolling around on their backs. Alanna noticed me gaping and wandered over to see what was going on. "*Ohmygodthey'resocute!*" Ellen and Kristen came running. Soon our whole family was crowded at the window watching the skunks play. They really were adorable. Whenever one of them strayed too far from the den's entrance their mother would shoo them back to safety. Once she even picked up one of the more adventurous babies by the scruff of his neck and carried him to the hole.

"Don't get too attached to them, girls," I warned. "The guy from the pest control company is coming in a couple of days with a trap to catch the mother. I'll have to call him back tomorrow to let him know there are babies now, too."

"They're not going to hurt them, are they, Dad?" the girls asked worriedly. "They're so cute!"

"I don't know what they do with skunks after they catch them. I'll find out when I call."

"Hi, my name's Donovan Gray. I called recently about getting rid of a skunk living under our front steps."

"Oh yeah, I remember. Name's Zeke. I'll be out with a trap first thing in the morning."

"There's been a new development – she had a bunch of babies. Can you catch them too?"

"Sure, no problem. Cost ya extra, though."

"That's okay. Listen, what do you do with them after they're caught?"

"Drown 'em."

"Oh."

"Somethin' wrong?"

"My kids have sort of bonded with the skunks, especially the babies. Can I pay extra to have them all released in a forest somewhere?"

"Nope."
"Why not?"
"Against comp'ny policy."
"Can you make an exception? I'll make it worth your while."
"Nope. Sorry. See ya tomorrow."

My daughters were at the window watching the octet play "sniff my bum" when I broke the bad news. They were crushed.

"We can't let him kill them, Dad! They're just babies! There has to be something we can do!" Tears welled up in their eyes. I'm a total sucker when it comes to tears.

"Okay, okay, I'll tell you what – we'll let him set the trap box for the mother, then when we've got her I'll catch the babies myself and set them all free in a forest."

"Huzzah!"

Zeke set up the trap a few feet from the den the following morning. It was basically a three-foot long rectangular box with an entrance at one end and a see-saw plank on the bottom. Sardines were placed at the far end. When the skunk smelled the bait and entered the box, her weight would make the plank tilt, which would then cause the trapdoor to slide down and seal the entrance. Somehow it seemed far too obvious to actually work.

"She'll never fall for it," I predicted confidently at supper that evening.

Around midnight Jan went out to investigate a rattling noise in the front yard. Sure enough, Skunky was caught in the trap.

The next morning was scorching hot and the weather geeks were forecasting a high of 32 degrees Celsius. I didn't want our new ward to die of heat exhaustion, so I decided to move the trap box to the shed in our backyard. After suiting up in a T-shirt, old jeans, coveralls, boots, goggles and a baseball cap, I tiptoed to the box and gingerly lifted it. I had envisioned her throwing a fit and spraying, but she remained calm. Once she was safely ensconced in the shed I went to the house and got some sardines and water. The trap box had a small latched opening on top that I presumed could be used to feed the animal inside. When I opened it, Skunky stuck her nose out and sniffed. It gave me quite a scare. I tossed the sardines in, poured her a cupful of water and hastily closed the latch.

I knew I had to catch the babies before their mother died in captivity. Every 30 minutes or so I went to the living room window to see if any of them had ventured out of the den. When I checked at noon they were all playing in the front yard. I ran to the garage and changed into my Captain Skunk costume. I then got a big plastic Rubbermaid storage bin and stealthily snuck up on the gallivanting brood. My plan was to drop the bin upside-down on top of them, thereby catching all or at least most of them in one fell swoop. I also figured that approach would minimize my chances of getting sprayed. Unfortunately, the little buggers hadn't read my memo that morning and they weren't playing in a tight rectangular formation. If I tried trapping them under the bin I'd only catch two or three at most, plus there was a high likelihood that at least one of them would get squashed by the rim.

I was standing on the lawn trying to come up with an alternate plan when one of baby skunks noticed me. To my surprise, she did a cartoony double-take and then squeaked a warning to the group. They all took one look in my direction and started running pell-mell for the den entrance. I lunged at them and managed to grab the last one just as she was about to escape down the hole. The poor thing was scared stiff. A small white spot near her bum area bulged. What in tarnation is that? *Poof!* Yecch! Sulphur-stink fart! I dropped her in the bin and placed it in the shed beside the trap box. I then put my skunk-catching outfit in the garage and took a very long shower.

The remaining skunks didn't show their faces for the rest of the day. When Jan and the kids got home at 4:30 that afternoon they all said: "Eeew! What's that horrible smell in the garage?"

I moved my skunk-wear from the garage to the shed.

I worked a graveyard shift that night. When I got home at 9:00 in the morning the first thing I did was feed Skunky and Slowpoke. After that I brought my bedding to the living room and set up shop on the sofa near the window so I'd be able to keep an eye on the den entrance. Whenever a skunk poked its little head out I'd put on my (increasingly stinky) duds and try to grab it. Most times I came back empty-handed, because they were getting smarter with each encounter. By the end of the day I considered myself lucky to have caught three more.

The following morning I went to feed the menagerie in the shed. The babies were fine, but Skunky hadn't touched her supper. When I shook the trap box there was no movement inside. The way the device was constructed it was impossible to see the animal within unless it happened to be sitting directly below the latched opening. I tried using a flashlight, but I still couldn't see her. Was she prone at the far end of the box, listlessly knocking on heaven's door? The babies wouldn't stand much of a chance if their mother died. I hurried back to my post in the living room.

By mid-afternoon I had captured the rest of the litter. I put them all in the trap box with their mother, rolled down every window in my truck and drove off in search of the closest backwoods. On my way out of town a police car pulled up beside me at a red light. If they caught a whiff of my exceedingly pungent vehicle they'd probably conclude I was some kind of deranged serial killer transporting body parts to the local dump. I whistled an Ozark Mountain banjo tune and tried to act casual.

Eventually I found a suitable location. It was a field adjacent to a medium-sized forest out in the middle of nowhere. I parked by the roadside and retrieved the box from the back of the truck. After hiking to the edge of the forest I put it on the ground and tied a 20-foot string to the trapdoor. I then yanked on the string from a safe distance and waited for the skunks to come tearing out. None of them emerged. I inched a bit closer and looked. The door was wide open. What was the problem? Surely they couldn't all have died during our drive out to the boonies.

I approached the box circumspectly and nudged it with my boot. Nothing. Crap! I picked it up and jiggled it forcefully. Skunky shot out like a bat out of hell and raced for the tree line. She stopped about 50 feet away and turned around to watch me warily. With one eye on Skunky, I gently shook the eight babies out. I took a few steps back and waited for them to trundle off to their mother. Instead, they all came to me. I backed away some more, but they continued following me and making mewling noises. Then it dawned on me. *They want me to feed them again!* I pulled the last tin of sardines out of my pocket, opened it and put the fish on the ground. Eight baby skunks huddled at my feet and had an early supper. While they were busy eating I picked up the trap box and walked to the truck. When I turned for one final look Skunky was strolling over to join her offspring.

For This I Went to Med School? *(Quiet Sméagol!)*

I call the 60 minutes between 2:00 and 3:00 a.m. the Jethro Hour. That's when the bars close and dozens of our city's brightest and best stagger out into the streets to engage in the time-honored tradition of nocturnal brawling. Once the punch-ups have concluded, the vanquished slowly make their way to the nearest ER to get their boo-boos fixed. It's *les gueules cassés*, Peg-style. Funny, but I can't seem to recall anyone mentioning this aspect of medicine during the Career Week lectures I attended in Grade 12. Stimulating work, saving lives, good pay: yes. Mangled drunks hurling on your shoes: no. Perhaps I nodded off during that part of the presentation.

A few nights ago I was working a shift at my regular ER. At about 2:00 a.m. the charge nurse handed me a chart and said, "Wait'll you see this guy!" Man, I hate it when she says that. Nine times out of 10 it ends up being something that makes me pine for early retirement. "Sorry I wasn't able to get much of a history," she continued. "His friend pretty much dragged him in, poured him onto the triage desk and took off. When I asked him what the big hurry was he said something about wanting to get back to the bar before last call." Ah, true loyalty. I went in to have a gander at my latest prize.

The patient dozing on the stretcher was a 25-year-old man in a Guns N' Roses T-shirt, disintegrating jeans and a pair of army boots several decades past their prime. An impressive array of contusions and abrasions covered his face. His brown, shoulder-length mullet was thoroughly caked with dried blood.

"Whoa, what happened to you?" I asked.

He opened his eyes, sat up groggily and gave me a lopsided grin.

"I have no idea, doc."

The facial contusions didn't look too bad, but he had four or five scalp lacerations that were going to require stitches. As I gathered my suturing paraphernalia I tried to jog his memory.

"What's the last thing you remember?"

"Pulling up to the bar in my buddy Dave's old beater. We finished off our road beers in the car before we went inside."

"And then . . . ?"

"Totally blank."

I gave him my patented Gregorian monk head shave and sutured the gashes on his scalp. He was a good sport about it. In fact, he monologued non-stop the entire time. After 20 minutes of listening to him rabbit on about his top-10 retro bands, his all-time favourite concert experiences and why stoned is so much more mellow than drunk, I turfed him down the hall to the radiology suite for a CT scan of his head.

Half an hour later he was back.

"Hey, doc, I can remember some more now!"

"Yes?"

"Inside the bar I got into a major argument with this guy over who was the greatest band of all time. I said obviously Guns N' Roses ruled, but he kept insisting it was Mötley Crüe. Can you believe that? What a moron!"

"Indeed. So, what happened next?"

"Not a clue."

An ambulance arrived with a patient in florid congestive heart failure. After dealing with that case I logged on to one of the diagnostic imaging computers and reviewed Amnesia Boy's CT scan. It looked fine. On my way past his room I popped in to give him a quick update.

"Good news – your scan's normal."

"Excellent! Rock on, dude! Hey, I remember even more now!"

"Yes?"

"Yeah, I remember me and Dave snuck out to the parking lot around 1:30 to have a little hoot of sinsemilla. It was, like, totally wicked, man!"

"Great. And then . . . ?"

"After we finished we looked up and saw the Crüe fanboy staring at us from across the parking lot."

"Uh-huh . . . ."

"He was holding a baseball bat."

I could see where this was heading.

"For some reason Dave took off, but I was kinda curious about something, so I jogged over to the guy to ask him a question."

"What did you ask him?"

"Hey dude, what's the bat for?"

So There You Have It, Folks

- A brief account of how a city slicker wound up becoming a denizen of the country. As you can probably tell, I thoroughly enjoyed rural living. For those of you who have never ventured beyond your city's perimeter for any prolonged period of time, perhaps you should consider giving it a try. You may be pleasantly surprised!

- A glimpse into the world of medicine and the mind of your average family physician and ER doc. Now you can almost hazard a guess as to what the person on the other end of the stethoscope is thinking. As you can see, it's generally something positive. Except when it isn't. JK!

- The tale of how Jan and I met, had three daughters, and raised them. Ellen is now 19, Kristen is 18 and Alanna is 17. As you can imagine, there's a whole lot of estrogen floating around in our house. Living with three teenage girls is a real challenge. Some days I feel like pulling my hair out! Oh, wait a minute – I have no hair . . . .

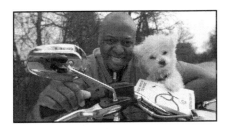

About the Author

Donovan Gray was born in Kingston, Jamaica, in 1962. After spending several years in Jamaica, Bermuda and Quebec, his family eventually moved to Winnipeg, Manitoba. Donovan has always enjoyed both writing and the sciences, and in 1983 he found himself having to make an unusual choice: honours English or medical school? In the end, he opted for the latter. In 1990 he graduated from the University of Manitoba with a degree in family and emergency medicine. After a year of ER work in Winnipeg he moved to rural Ontario to start a practice, and shortly thereafter, a family.

In 2004 Donovan, his wife Janet and their three daughters heeded the call of extended family and returned to Winnipeg. He is currently a full-time ER physician. Once the north gets in your blood it's hard to get it out, though, so he continues to do regular locums in northern Ontario.

Donovan has contributed medical short stories to the *Medical Post* as well as the *National Post*. Front-running titles for his next book are *Night of the Living Jethros* and *Mamas, Don't Let Your Babies Grow Up to Be ER Docs*. He also hasn't ruled out *Fifty Years of Gray!*

www.dudewheresmystethoscope.ca

Manufactured by Amazon.ca
Bolton, ON

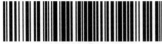
10555681R00125